Oral and Maxillofacial Surgery

Edited by Gokul Sridharan

Published in London, United Kingdom

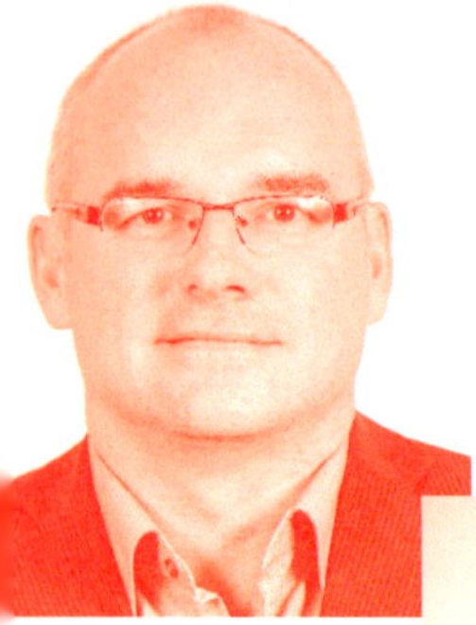
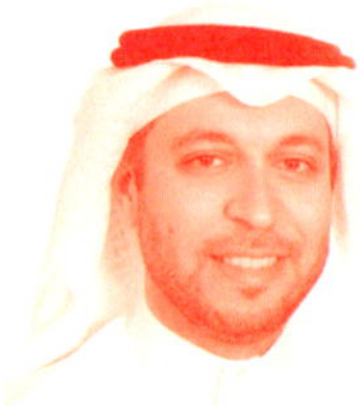
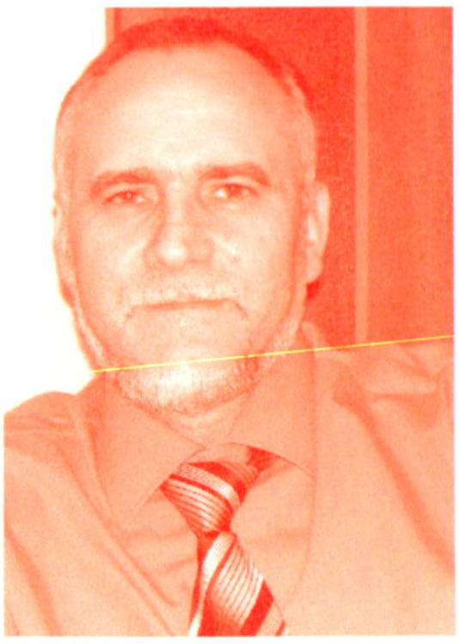
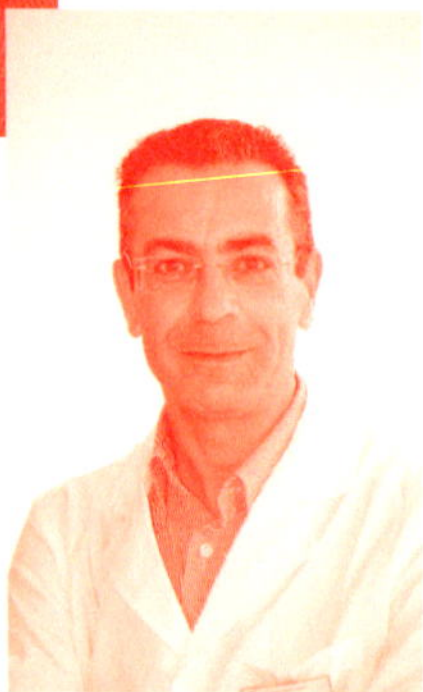
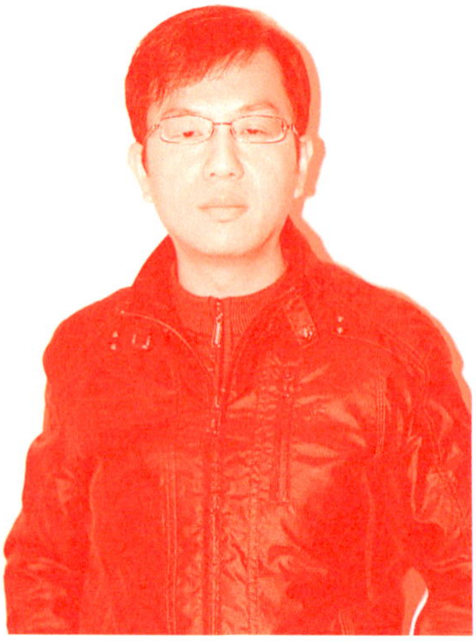
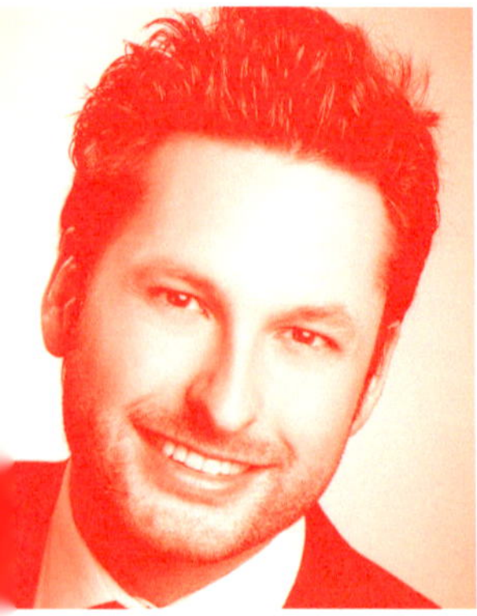
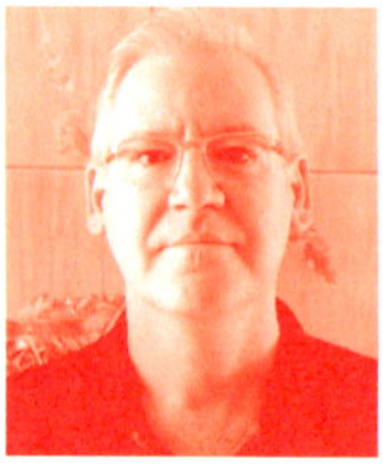

IntechOpen

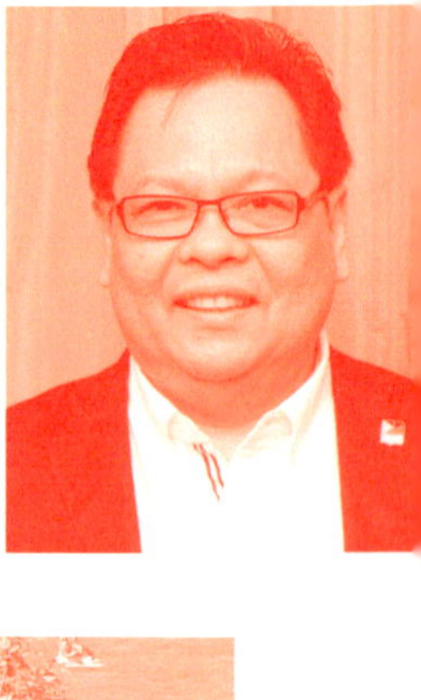
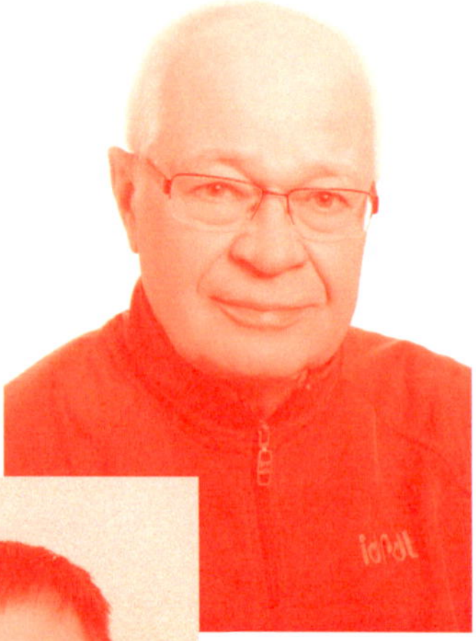
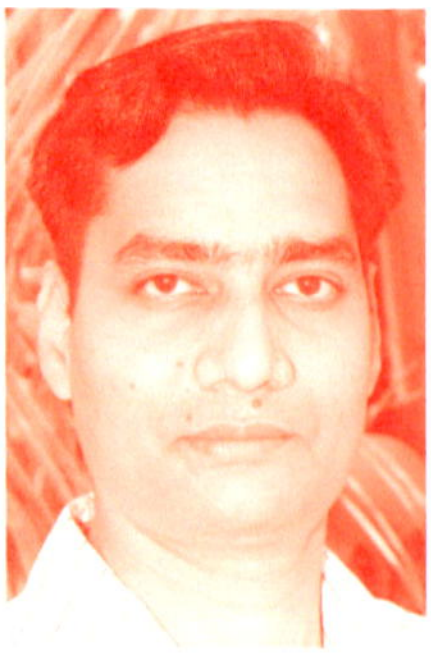
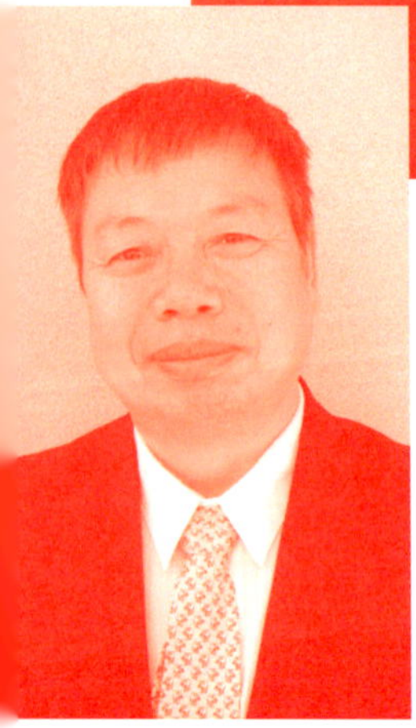
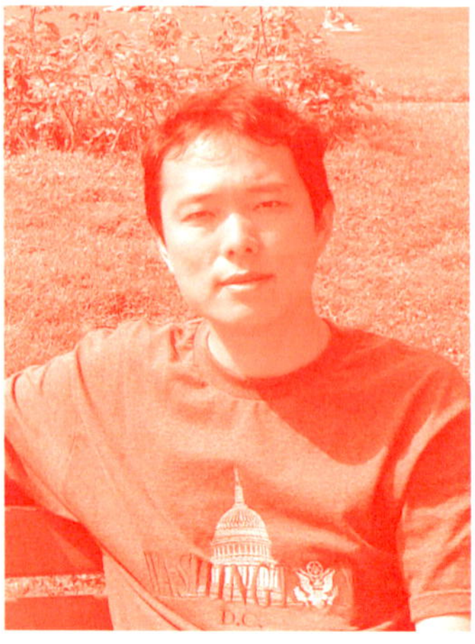
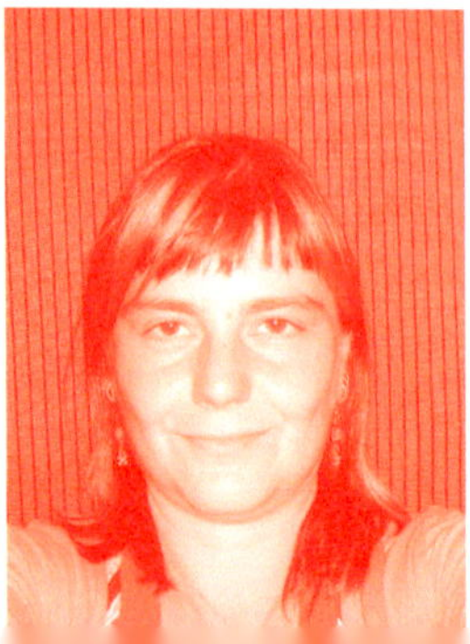

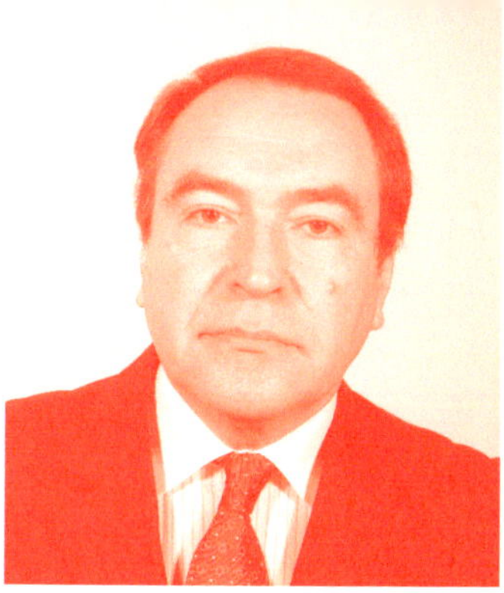
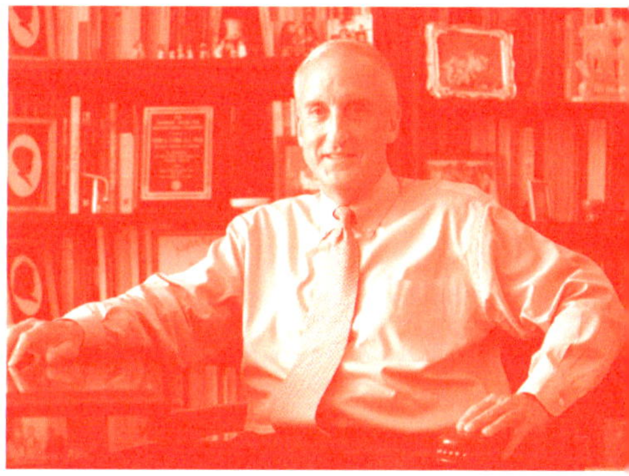
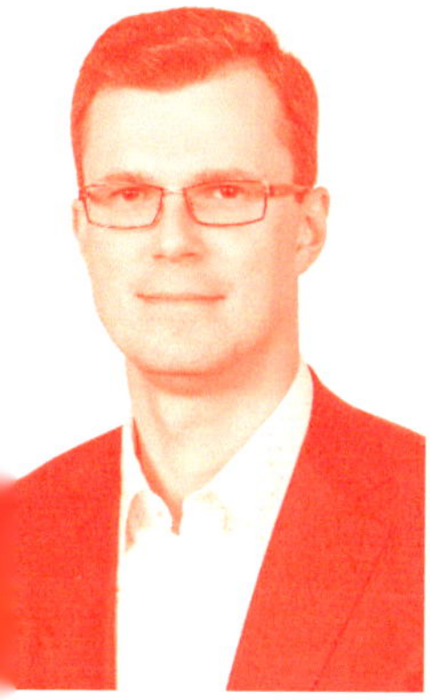
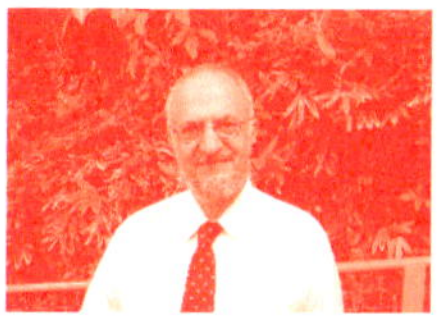
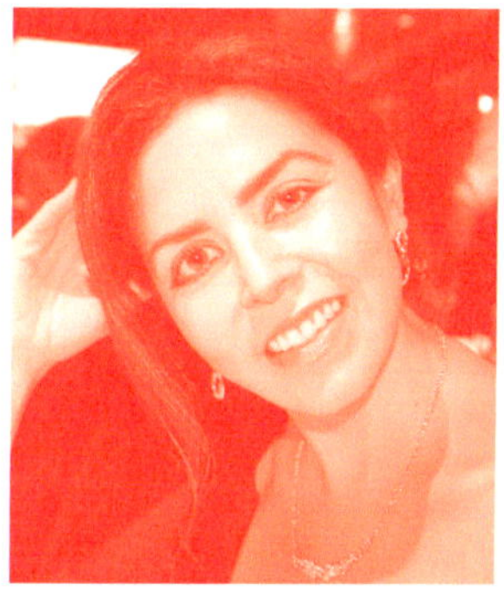

Supporting open minds since 2005

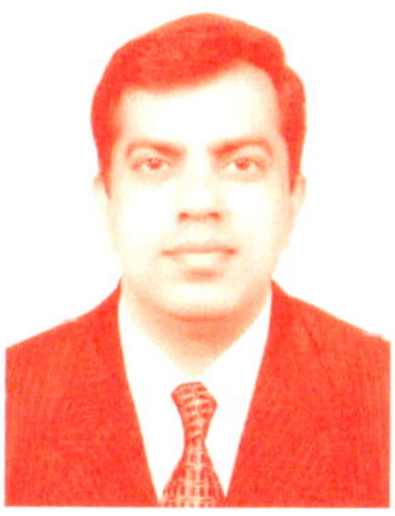
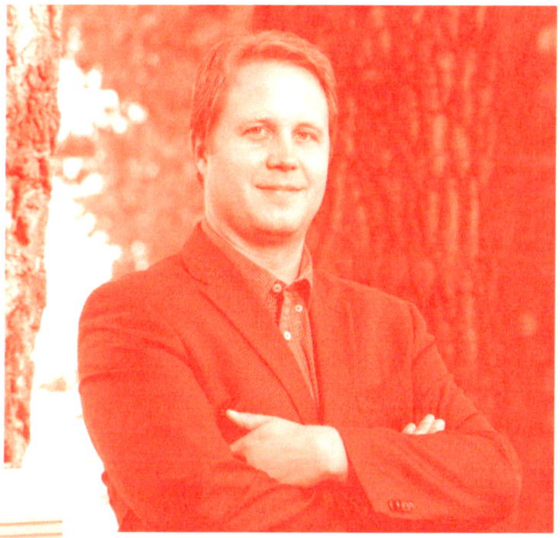
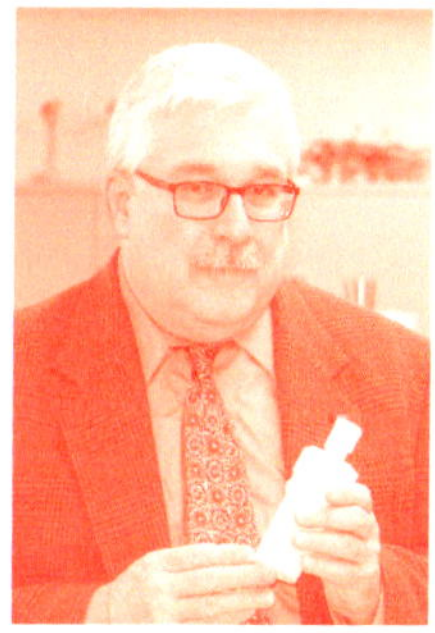
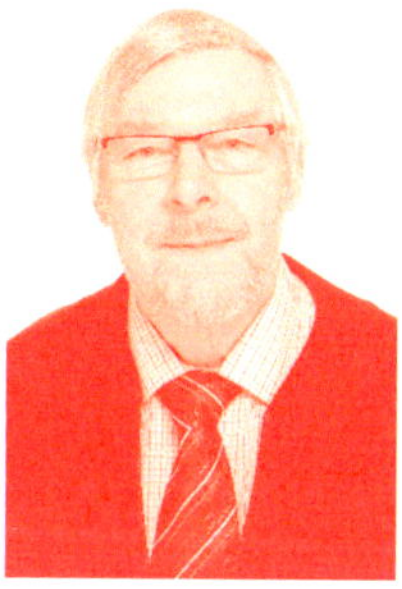
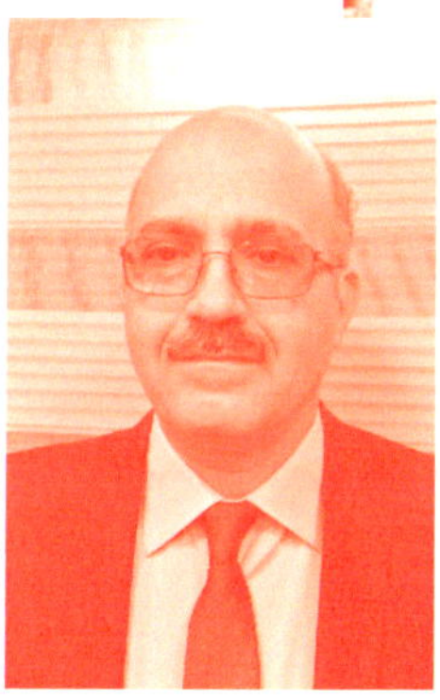
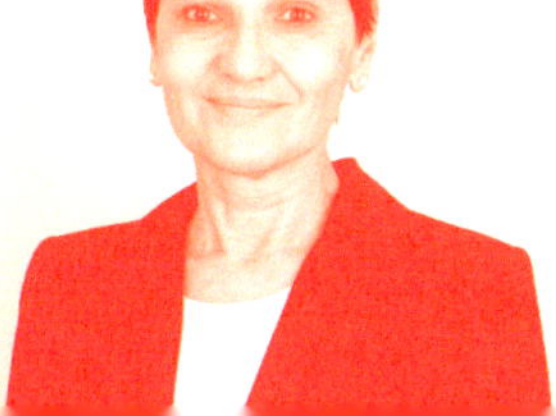
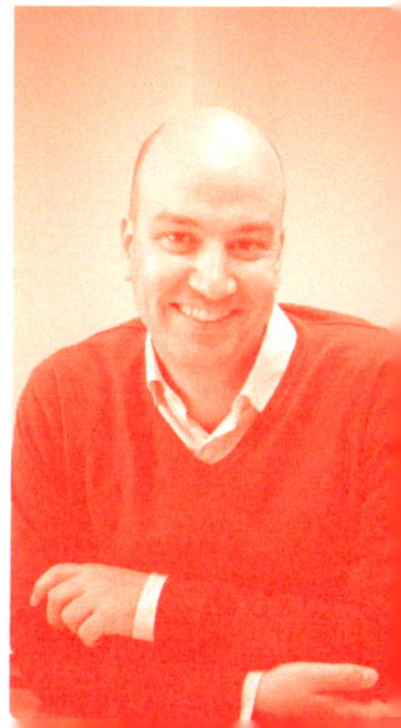

Oral and Maxillofacial Surgery
http://dx.doi.org/10.5772/intechopen.87318
Edited by Gokul Sridharan

Contributors
Omar Sheikh, Matin Madadian, Amanveer Benning, Aynur Emine Cicekcibasi, Gülay Acar, Krishna Sireesha Sundaragiri, Soumya Makarla, Bharat Sankhla, Tina Nazerani, Reingard M. Aigner, Peter Kalmar, Melike Aytekin, Volkan Arisan, Leandro Díez Suárez, Antonio Gómez Pedraza, Vicente González Cardín, Martín Granados García, Kasi Ganesh Sriraam, K. Rajendran Arun Vignesh, Onur Gonul, Ahmet Usame Çiçek, Onur Atalı, Faysal Uğurlu, Murat Afat

First published in London, United Kingdom, 2021 by IntechOpen
IntechOpen is the global imprint of INTECHOPEN LIMITED, registered in England and Wales, registration number: 11086078, 5 Princes Gate Court, London, SW7 2QJ, United Kingdom
Printed in Croatia

British Library Cataloguing-in-Publication Data
A catalogue record for this book is available from the British Library

Additional hard and PDF copies can be obtained from orders@intechopen.com

Oral and Maxillofacial Surgery
Edited by Gokul Sridharan
p. cm.
Print ISBN 978-1-83880-335-3
Online ISBN 978-1-83880-336-0
eBook (PDF) ISBN 978-1-83880-460-2

For EU product safety concerns:
IN TECH d.o.o., Prolaz Marije Krucifikse Kozulić 3, 51000 Rijeka, Croatia, info@intechopen.com or visit our website at intechopen.com.

Meet the editor

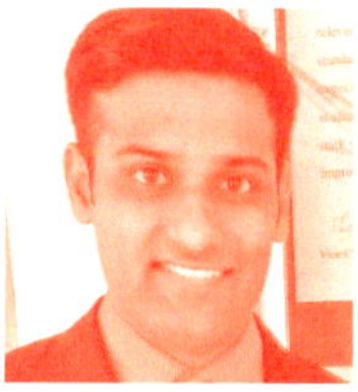

Dr. Gokul Sridharan is currently an associate professor in the Department of Oral Pathology and Microbiology at Y.M.T. Dental College and Hospital, Navi Mumbai. He obtained his Ph.D. for the work titled "Salivary and serum metabolomics in oral leukoplakia and oral squamous cell carcinoma." His fields of interest include oral pre-cancer, oral cancer, salivary diagnostics, oral and maxillofacial diseases, and advanced diagnostic aids with an emphasis on bioinformatics and metabolomics. He has several scientific publications to his credit and actively contributes as a peer reviewer to numerous journals. He is an active member of the editorial boards of several journals of repute. Dr. Sridharan has undergone training and is a qualified diploma holder in medical law and ethics and is certified in tobacco cessation and control as well.

Contents

Preface

Oral and maxillofacial surgery is a specialized branch of dentistry that deals with the surgical management of various head and neck pathologies. The specialty focuses on reconstructive surgery of the oro-facial region, surgery of facial trauma, the oral cavity and jaws, dental implants as well as cosmetic surgery. Certain head and neck pathologies routinely encountered that require surgical intervention include maxillofacial trauma, odontogenic cysts and tumors, and head and neck malignancies, among others. The objectives of surgical procedures in this field are to remove any pathology, maintain post-operative aesthetics, and prevent a recurrence. Over the years, oral and maxillofacial surgery has undergone major modifications with increased emphasis on tissue preservation and maintenance of normal anatomy and functions of the oro-facial tissues. In addition to the surgical treatment of the head and neck pathologies, oral and maxillofacial surgery is also involved in dental implants and various cosmetic surgeries. The head and neck anatomy is characterized by a complex network of neural and vascular systems and consists of an extensive lymphatic supply. Hence, it is imperative that oral and maxillofacial surgeons have an extensive understanding of head and neck anatomy to aid them in better treatment planning and execution. This book presents an overview of head and neck anatomy and discusses recent concepts associated with different surgical procedures. It provides surgeons in this field with updated information on current surgical trends and their applications.

Dr. Gokul Sridharan MDS, PhD, PGD (Medical Law and Ethics)
Associate Professor,
Department of Oral Pathology and Microbiology,
Dr. G. D. Pol Foundation,
YMT Dental College and Hospital,
Kharghar, Navi Mumbai, India

Section 1

Basics of Oral and Maxillofacial Surgery

Chapter 1

Surgical Anatomy of the Temporal Bone

Gülay Açar and Aynur Emine Çiçekcibaşı

Abstract

Numerous neurological lesions and tumors of the paranasal sinuses and oral cavity may spread into the middle and posterior cranial fossae through the anatomical apertures. For the appropriate management of these pathologies, many extensive surgical approaches with a comprehensive overview of the anatomical landmarks are required from the maxillofacial surgery's point of view. The surgical significance lies in the fact that iatrogenic injury to the petrous segment of the temporal bone including the carotid artery, sigmoid sinus, and internal jugular vein, can lead to surgical morbidity and postoperative pseudoaneurysm, vasospasm, or carotid-cavernous fistula. To simplify understanding complex anatomy of the temporal bone, we aimed to review the surgical anatomy of the temporal bone focusing on the associations between the surface landmarks and inner structures. Also, breaking down an intricate bony structure into smaller parts by compartmental approach could ease a deep concentration and navigation. To identify the anatomic architecture of the temporal bone by using reference points, lines and compartments can be used to supplement anatomy knowledge of maxillofacial surgeons and may improve confidence by surgical trainees. Especially, this systematic method may provide an easier way to teach and learn surgical spatial structure of the petrous pyramid in clinical applications.

Keywords: maxillofacial surgery, segmentation, surface landmarks, surgical anatomy, temporal bone

1. Introduction

The temporal bone is a dense complex bone that constitutes the lower lateral aspect of the skull and has complex anatomy because of the three-dimensional relationships between neurovascular structures. The petrous portion of the temporal bone has a role as the partition between the middle and posterior cranial fossae. It articulates with the occipital bone (occipitomastoid suture) posteriorly, the parietal bone (squamous suture) superiorly, the sphenoid bone (spheno-squamosal suture) and the zygomatic bone (arcus zygomaticus) anteriorly, and the mandible (temporomandibular joint) inferiorly [1, 2]. It contains multiple intrinsic channels, along with the internal carotid artery (ICA), cranial nerves, and sigmoid sinus (SS), all within intricate spatial architecture. Owing to a complex web of foramina and neurovascular structures of the temporal bone, the lateral skull base is a technically difficult region for surgeons. Because the middle and inner ear structures of hearing and equilibrium are preserved in the temporal bone, a surgical dissection of it requires thorough understanding of three-dimensional (3D) map of the topographic anatomy to avoid iatrogenic risks. The relationship between the surface landmarks and expected internal structures and the segmentation of the temporal structures by using key surgical lines and spaces allow a better understanding of its anatomic architecture. Each temporal bone consists of five distinct osseous segments including the squamous, tympanic, petrous, mastoid, and styloid portions [3, 4].

2. External anatomy of the temporal portions

2.1 The squamous portion

The anterosuperior part of the temporal bone is a large flattened scale-like plate that forms the lateral boundary of the middle cranial fossa. It has three borders and two surfaces [1].

2.1.1 Borders and surfaces of the squamous portion

Superiorly, it overlaps the sculpted squamous margin of the middle third of the parietal bone and constructs the squamosal suture. Posteriorly, it forms the occipitomastoid suture with the squamous part of the occipital bone. Also, there is an angle, parietal notch, between the squamous and mastoid portions of the temporal bone (**Figure 1**). Antero-inferiorly, its thick serrated margin takes part in pterion formation and articulates with the greater wing of the sphenoid bone to form the spheno-squamosal suture. Inferiorly, it fuses and forms the petro-squamous suture with the superior surface of the petrous portion by extending medially as tegmen tympany [5, 6].

External surface, the greater part of the temporal fossa, provides origin to the temporalis muscle and is limited below by the curved line, the temporal line, that lies from the supra-meatal crest to the mastoid cortex posteriorly. Below this line, just above and behind the external acoustic meatus (EAM), the supra-meatal triangle (Macewen's triangle) contains the supra-meatal spine, spine of Henle and the cribriform area (**Figure 1**). Also, the squamo-mastoid suture is located approximately 1 cm below the temporal line [5–7]. On this smooth surface, there is a sulcus for the middle temporal artery, which is the medial branch of the superficial temporal artery (STA). Antero-inferiorly, the zygomatic process projects by two roots: the upper border of the posterior root forms the supra-meatal crest and the lower border forms a laterally based projection, known as post-glenoid tubercle or process (PGP). Inferiorly, the concavity along the surface of the anterior root is called the glenoid fossa (GF), which is bounded by the articular eminence (ArE) anteriorly and the PGP posteriorly [5–7].

Internal surface is rough and concave in shape, and the anterior and posterior divisions of middle meningeal artery (MMA) run in a groove on this surface that defines the boundary of middle cranial fossa with impressions for the gyri of the temporal lobe. Inferiorly, it forms the petro-squamosal suture with the anterior surface of the petrous part [5, 6].

2.1.2 Surgical landmarks and ossification of the squamous portion

The Macewen's triangle, a surgical surface marking for the mastoid antrum (MA), is formed between the temporal line superiorly, the posterosuperior wall of the EAM antero-inferiorly, and the opening of the mastoid emissary vein or

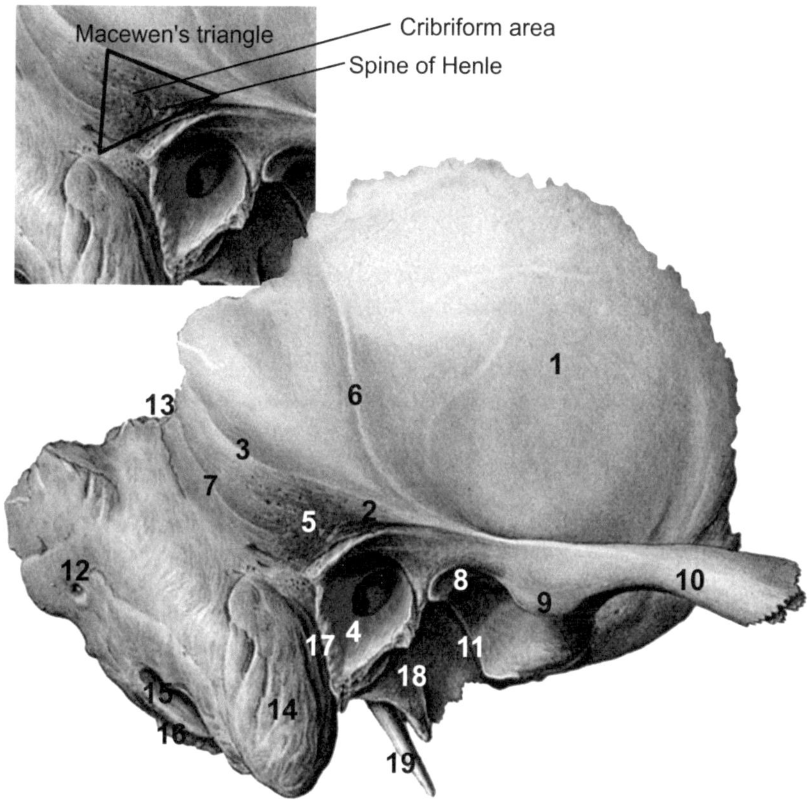

Figure 1.
The surface landmarks on the squamous portion: 1, temporal fossa; 2, supra-meatal crest; 3, temporal line; 4, external acoustic meatus; 5, supra-meatal triangle (Macewen's triangle); 6, middle temporal artery; 7, squamo-mastoid suture; 8, mandibular fossa (glenoid fossa); 9, articular eminence; 10, zygomatic process; 11, petrotympanic fissure (Glaserian fissure); 12, mastoid foramen; 13, parietal notch; 14, mastoid process; 15, mastoid notch (digastric fossa); 16, occipital sulcus; 17, tympano-mastoid suture; 18, vaginal process; 19, styloid process.

sinodural angle posteriorly (**Figure 1**). The temporal line corresponds to the tegmen tympani (TT), which is a bony plate below the middle cranial fossa dura and over the mastoid air cells. The mastoid cortex posterior to the spine of Henle is a guide to the lateral wall of the MA and located 15 mm deep to it in adults but in new born about 2 mm [5, 6, 8]. The cribriform area in Macewen's triangle is perforated by numerous small holes that serve as a passage for the vessels of the mucosa of the antrum. The dissection along the margins of this triangle is safer because the vital neurovascular structures are absent. Peris-Celda et al. reported that the temporal line is supratentorial and infratentorial in 93% and 7% of the cases, respectively [9]. During retro-auricular mastoidectomy, the MA may be exposured by drilling the cribriform area and provides a safer surgical approach to the tympanic cavity. The tympanic portion and the styloid process may show variations depending on the shape and the position of the spine of Henle. The MA is located in the same line of the spine of Henle at about 10 years; then the MA is enlarged and placed 1 cm behind it [6, 9].

The MMA lies underneath the pterion which is a common junction between the temporal, parietal, frontal, and sphenoid bones. The fracture of this weakest bony part may result in an epidural bleeding. Between the temporal muscle and fascia, the STA and the superficial temporal vein (STV) courses in close proximity with the zygomaticotemporal (ZTN) and the auriculotemporal (ATN) nerves, branches of the trigeminal nerve (TN). Because of a vessel running superficial to the nerve (80% STA), the underlying nerve may be compressed and results in temporal migraine headache. Lee et al. reported that the intersection (compression) point among the ATN, STA, and STV was at an average of 40 mm superior and 10 mm anterior to the tragus, which is a significant surface landmark at the most anterosuperior point of the EAM. The applications of surgical decompression of the ATN in these compression points improve migraine headache [10].

The anterior articular part of the GF is formed by a gentle sloped area of the squamous portion, which facilitates the movement of the temporomandibular joint (TMJ) during wide mouth opening. At the lateral aspect of the ArE, a small bony ridge, articular tubercle (AT), serves as an attachment for the lateral collateral ligament. The PGP inhibits backward displacement of mandibular head and participates to the superior wall of the EAM [8]. The posterior nonarticular part of the GP is formed by the tympanic portion and the squamo-tympanic suture intervenes between them. The inferior edge of the TT (petrous part) divides this suture into two: a petro-squamosal fissure in front and a petrotympanic fissure (Glaserian fissure) behind (**Figure 1**). The chorda tympani nerve, a branch of the facial nerve, exits the temporal bone through the Glaserian fissure and joins the lingual nerve as the parasympathetic input to start the submandibular and sublingual gland secretions [2, 4, 5].

The articulation between the GF and the condyle of the mandible is called TMJ, which plays an essential role in speech, respiration, swallowing, and specially mastication. Because the TMJ is in close proximity with the MMA, some surgical landmarks around the TMJ and foramen spinosum (FS) play a critical role in surgical approaches. Miller et al. reported that researchers measured the distances from the zygomatic root (first projection of the zygomatic arch = PGP) to some surgical landmarks such as the arcuate eminence (AE), the head of the malleus (HM) under the TT, and the FS to identify the location of the internal auditory meatus (IAM) or the superior semicircular canal (SSC). Also, they described the superior petrosal triangle as a consistent triangle between the zygomatic root, the FR, and the HM to localize the bony tegmen over the tympanic cavity [11]. Baur et al. offered simply identifiable reference landmarks including the AE, the most lateral aspect of the Glaserian fissure and the FS and measured the distances between them to predict the location of the MMA [12]. According to these researchers, the internal landmarks including the HM and Bill's bar (the vertical crest in the fundus of the internal auditory canal) are in a single plane with the zygomatic root [11].

After the ArE forming the anterior limit of the GF, the anterior root continues in front as a bony ridge that forms the posterior boundary of the infratemporal fossa, which is a small triangular area transmitting the neurovascular structures between the pterygopalatine fossa and temporal fossa. Then, a serrated anterior end of the zygomatic process passes straight forward and articulates with the temporal process of the zygomatic bone and completes the zygomatic arch. The temporal fascia inserts to this arch and the temporal line superiorly and also the masseter muscle origins from the arch inferiorly. The lateral temporomandibular ligament attaches to the AT, and the GF is covered with an articular disc to construct the synovial TMJ with the condyle of the mandible [5–7].

Anteriorly, the small part of squamous portion takes part in the infratemporal fossa formation with the zygomatic bone and the greater wing of the sphenoid bone. Below the zygomatic bone, the branches of the first and second mandibular parts of the MA with veins and the pterygoid plexus of veins, the mandibular and lingual nerves pass through the infratemporal fossa. During the infratemporal fossa approaching for surgical removal of tumors localized in the orbit, the maxillary and sphenoid sinuses, the detailed anatomical knowledge of these neurovascular structures is needed. Depending on the position of the infratemporal fossa below the floor of the middle cranial fossa and posterior to the maxilla, it is in close proximity with the parapharyngeal and masticator spaces. The parapharyngeal carotid artery enters the carotid canal (CC) behind the FS and foramen ovale. During transpterygoid infratemporal fossa approach, the positions of these surgical landmarks can be used to prevent ICA injury [13].

Ossification of the squamous portion starts intramembranously from one center around the zygomatic process at the 2nd month. At birth it fuses with the other membranous bone, tympanic portion. Normally, at birth the temporal bone consists of three parts; the petrous, squamous, and the tympanic [1].

2.2 The mastoid portion

The mastoid portion forms the pneumatized thick posterior part of the temporal bone. It fuses with the squamous portion antero-superiorly and the tympanic portion anteriorly and the petrous portion anteromedially. It has three borders and two surfaces [5, 6].

2.2.1 Borders and surfaces of the mastoid portion

Posteriorly, it articulates with the squamous part of the occipital bone between lateral angle and the jugular process and constructs the occipitomastoid suture. Inferiorly, the mastoid process extends as a rough and conical shaped projection and filled with mastoid cells variable in shape and size. Anteriorly, it associates with the tympanic portions of the temporal bone to form the tympano-mastoid suture, and the inferior auricular branch of the vagus nerve (Arnold's nerve) exits through this suture [5, 14, 15].

Near the squamo-mastoid suture, the occipital belly of occipito-frontalis and auricularis posterior muscles attach on the external surface that is perforated by numerous small foramina. At the posterior border of the mastoid portion or the occipitomastoid suture, the largest one, mastoid foramen is located and transmits an emissary vein connecting the SS with the posterior auricular vein and a branch of occipital artery to the dura mater (**Figure 1**). The mastoid process serves for the attachment of the sternocleidomastoid, splenius capitis, and longissimus capitis muscles and shows variations in shape and size with respect to sex. The posterior belly of the digastric muscle is originated from the mastoid notch (digastric fossa), which is a depression on the inferomedial margin of the mastoid process (**Figure 1**). More medial to the notch lies a sulcus, the occipital sulcus, forming a groove for the occipital artery [4, 6].

The internal surface includes a well-defined and curved sigmoid sulcus lying along its junction with the posterior surface of petrous part and lodges the SS, partially the transverse sinus, which are separated from mastoid air cells by a thin plate of bone. The mastoid foramen transmitting the mastoid emissary vein may be open to this sulcus. The SS begins as the continuation of the transverse sinus and lies downward in a S-shaped groove and opens into the superior jugular bulb. There is a sinodural angle between the dura plates of the SS and middle and posterior cranial fossae [2, 5, 9, 16].

2.2.2 Surgical landmarks and ossification of the mastoid portion

The mastoid process shows tree types of pneumatization patterns including pneumatic (full air cell), sclerotic (solid mass of bone), and mixed (air cells and bone marrow) types. Especially, in the anterosuperior part of the mastoid process, there is an irregular cavity that is larger than other mastoid cells and called MA, which corresponds to the cribriform area. It is covered with the mucous membrane of the tympanic cavity and communicates anteriorly with the epitympanic recess of the middle ear via the aditus ad antrum. The tegmen antri, a roof of the MA, separates it from the middle cranial fossa. During embryonic period, the squamous and petrous portions fused each other and forms the petro-squamous suture. In adults, it forms a thin bony septum, the Körner's septum, by extending into the mastoid process [1, 4, 6, 9, 17]. Körner's septum divides the mastoid air cells in the mastoid process into a deep petrous part medially and a superficial squamous part laterally. The petro-squamosal sinus or the mastoid emissary vein may infrequently be observed along this septum. During mastoidectomy or transmastoid approaches, awareness of this crucial landmark and its variations is essential to avoid iatrogenic complications. The squamous part starts to develop at 8th week, whereas the petrous part develops later at 6th months during embryogenesis, and each part opens into the MA separately [1]. Also, the mastoid cells are separated by bony plates from the adjacent structures such as the posterior wall of the EAM anteriorly, tegmen plate superiorly, SS posteriorly, digastric ridge inferiorly, and the lateral semicircular canal (LSC) or solid triangle medially. The solid triangle is a compact bony angle between three SCs. During the mastoidectomy, all the air cells around this septum and adjacent bony structures should be removed without damaging the bony plates. To avoid iatrogenic injury to the adjacent structures, the MA must be open superiorly toward TT. The tympano-mastoid suture at the posterior wall of the MA is surface marking of the course of the vertical portion of the facial nerve (FN) [9, 16, 18]. Peris-Celda et al. reported that the parietal notch corresponds to the posterior petrosal point and the SS (the transverse-SS junction) in 66 and 34% of the cases, respectively [9].

Ossification of the mastoid portion is endochondral which is identical to the petrous and styloid portions. At birth, the mastoid process is absent, and the MA is invisible and covered by a thin bony plate that is extension of the squamous portion. At the first year, the mastoid process becomes prominent and the petro-squamous suture arises. The antrum can be seen obviously at about the fifth year. During puberty, the thickness of the process increases, and it becomes pneumatic that is lined by mucous membrane. In adults, the mastoid process may not contain air cells in 20% cases [1, 2, 17].

2.3 The tympanic portion

An annular shaped part of the temporal bone forms the tympano-mastoid suture posteriorly and the squamo-tympanic suture superiorly (**Figure 1**). Medially, it fuses with the petrous portion, whereas a free lateral part of it constructs the major part of the EAM and also serves an attachment for the cartilaginous part of the external auditory canal (EAC). Its inferior margin is free, and it has two parts on the lateral surface; posterosuperior part forms the EAM, and anteroinferior part limits the mandibular fossa posteriorly [5, 19].

2.3.1 Borders and surfaces of the tympanic portion

Medially, just above the GF, this suture is subdivided by a thin tegmen part of the petrous portion into two: the petrotympanic fissure posteriorly and the petro-squamosal fissure anteriorly. Lateral part of this upper margin fuses with the back of the PGP to form the nonarticular part of the GF. Inferiorly, the lateral part of the margin gives an attachment for the deep part of the parotid fascia and forms the vaginal process, which wraps the root of the styloid process laterally [2, 4].

Laterally, external surface is bounded by the cartilaginous part of the EAC which extends from the auricle to the tympanic membrane. The EAC is an S-shaped tube, about 2.5 cm in long, that is composed of the lateral third cartilaginous part and the medial two-thirds osseous part [14, 15, 18]. The tympanic part constructs the anterior wall and floor and the lower part of posterior wall of the EAM, whereas the squamous part forms the superior and upper part of the posterior wall of it (**Figure 1**). The tympanic part grows from the tympanic ring, which is open U-shaped possessing two edge anterior and posterior. The anterior edge forms the tympano-squamous fissure within the anterosuperior part of the EAM and the petrotympanic fissure within the middle ear, whereas the posterior edge forms the tympano-mastoid fissure within the posteroinferior part of the EAM near the stylomastoid foramen (SMF) [2, 4, 19].

The internal surface fuses with the petrous portion and forms the tympanic sulcus for the lodgement of the tympanic membrane, which forms an angle about 55° with the floor of the EAM and separates the external and middle ear (ME). At the upper part, the tympanic sulcus does not fuse each other by forming the greater and lesser tympanic spines and a notch called Rivinus between them. This notch is closed by the pars flaccida of the tympanic membrane. The notch of Rivinus corresponds to the junction between the squamous and tympanic portions [1, 4, 14, 20].

2.3.2 Surgical landmarks and ossification of the tympanic portion

Ossification starts from the four centers around the tympanic ring at the end of the embryonic period (8th week) via intramembranous ossification of the EAM. The tympanic ring at first is nearly straight and then turns into horseshoe shape (annular) and then, the open arms extending upwards terminate in a notch for the location of the tympanic membrane between them. After birth, the upper segment of the tympanic bone grows rapidly but because of the gradual development of the lower segment, a deep notch (tympanic foramen) is left in the anterior part of the bony EAM. Normally, the tympanic ring fuses until the age of 5 year but a dehiscence may persist (range 4.6–22.7%) at the anteroinferior aspect of the EAM, called foramen of Huschke (foramen tympanicum). This fusion defect is not a true foramen, but it may cause a connection between the EAM and the posteromedial part of the TMJ and results in TMJ herniation and the secretion of the parotid gland and also the dissemination of tumor and infections into the EAM [1, 14, 19, 20]. Anteriorly, the EAM may communicate with the retromandibular part of the parotid gland via the fissures of Santorini within the anterior cartilage. Peris-Celda et al. reported that the SSC dehiscence can be observed approximately 1.5 cm posterior to the middle point of the EAM in 86% of the cases [9]. In newborn, the tympanic membrane is infiltrated with air and the tympanic ring forms a bony plate, which may cause the development of a cleft, the auricular fissure, posteriorly and a cleft, the tympano-squamous fissure, anteriorly [19, 20].

2.4 The petrous portion

The petrous portion is a dense pyramid-shaped bone and composed of the labyrinth of the internal ear, the tympanic cavity of the middle ear and a bony part of the auditory Eustachian tube (ET), and canals for the passage of the ICA and the FN. It is ossified from the otic capsule by forming a 45° angle with the horizontal axis. It has a base, an apex, and three surfaces and three borders [3, 4, 21].

2.4.1 Borders of the petrous portion

Superiorly, the petrous ridge is the longest border and a boundary between the posterior part of the middle cranial fossa (the anterior surface of the petrous part) and the anterior part of the posterior cranial fossa (the posterior surface of the petrous part). It contains a groove that lodges the superior petrosal sinus (SPS) and the lateral margin of tentorium cerebelli attaches to this margin (**Figure 2**). Posteriorly, the medial part of the posterior margin articulates with the basilar part of occipital bone along the petro-clival fissure and forms a groove that lodges the inferior petrosal sinus (IPS) that extends from the posteroinferior part of the cavernous sinus to the internal jugular vein (IJV). The lateral part of the posterior margin is free and limits the jugular foramen (JF) supero-laterally and has a triangular notch for the lodgement of the inferior ganglion of the glossopharyngeal

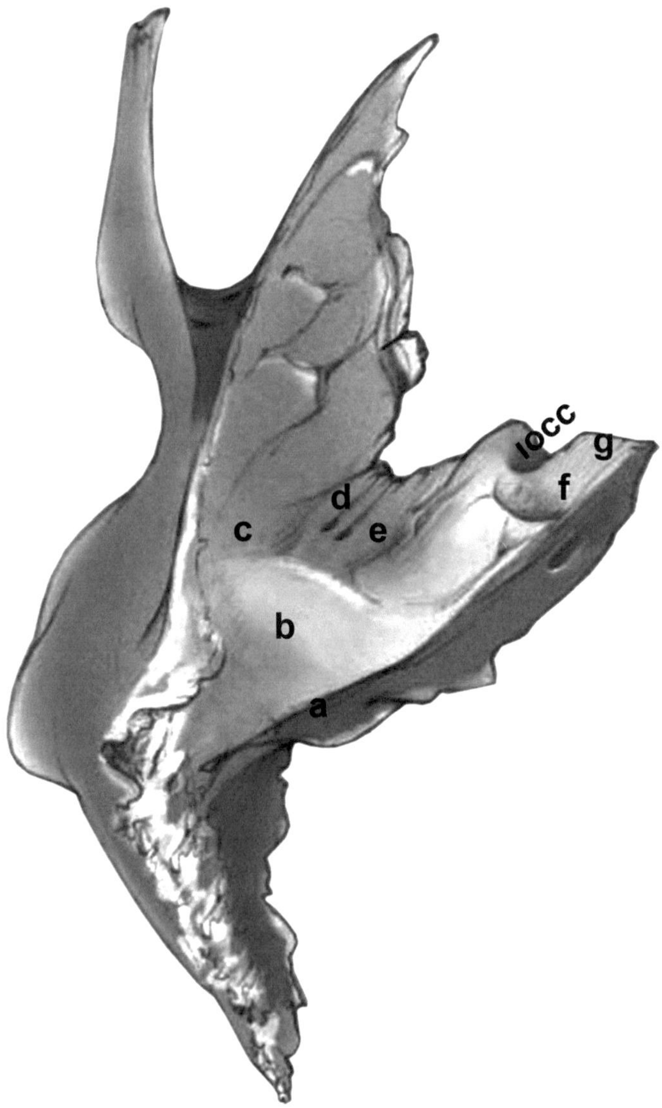

Figure 2.
The surface landmarks on the anterior surface of the petrous portion: a, petrous ridge (sulcus of the superior petrosal sinus); b, arcuate eminence; c, tegmen tympani; d, sulcus of the lesser petrosal nerve; e, sulcus of the greater petrosal nerve; f, trigeminal impression; g, petrous apex; iocc, internal opening of carotid canal.

nerve (Jacobson's nerve = GPN). Anterolateral border is formed by the ET extending from the anteroinferior wall of the tympanic cavity to the nasopharynx [3, 4, 9].

The base is integrated with the inner surface of the squamous and mastoid portions, whereas the apex forms the posterolateral margin of the foramen lacerum (FL) and faces the Meckel's cave medially. There is a fibrocartilage connection between the apex and the clivus. The internal opening of the carotid canal (IOCC) is observed at the apex for the intracranial entry of the ICA. At the anterolateral part of the FL, the petro-sphenoid ligament connects the tip of the apex to the dorsum sellae of the sphenoid and the abducent nerve lies below this ligament and enters the cavernous sinus adjoining the ICA [1, 7, 16].

2.4.2 Surgical landmarks on the anterior surface of the petrous portion

Anterior surface describes a triangular area, between the linear lines as follows: a horizontal line that starts from the preauricular burrhole in front of the tragus to petrous apex at the FL and passes through the FS anteriorly, the petrous ridge posteriorly and the petro-squamous suture, which lies along the junction of the petrous pyramid with the vertical part of the squamous portion laterally [3, 16, 22]. It consists of some marking landmarks (**Figure 2**).

a. The anteromedial two-third of the musculotubal canal is cartilaginous, whereas the posterolateral third is bony. The bony part consists of two small canals that are separated by a thin bony septum at the lateral part the petrous portion. The tensor tympani muscle passes through the superior semicanal, whereas the inferior semicanal forms the bony portion of the ET. The tensor tympani muscle originates from the greater wing of the sphenoid and inserts into the upper part of the medial surface of the handle of malleus after making a bend around the processus cochleariformis in the tympanic cavity [4, 6]. The ET lies between the tympanic orifice and the isthmus, which has the smallest diameter at the intersection point of the petrous and squamous parts of the temporal bone just behind the sphenoid spine. Brown et al. reported that the ET is subdivided by genu within the membranocartilaginous part into two portions; posterior horizontal ET between the genu and the anterior attachment of the tympanic membrane ridge, whereas the anterior vertical ET lies from the genu to the nasopharyngeal orifice and opens into the nasopharynx. During endoscopic eustachian tube obliteration, the ET is cannulated to treat refractory CSF rhinorrhea by identifying three anatomic parameters: the ET length, isthmus diameter, and genu location. According to a new surgical classification, the cartilaginous portion of the ET is divided into the petrous, lacerum, pterygoid, and nasopharyngeal parts. The bony part attaches to the ET sulcus or sulcus tuba, which is contiguous to the FL medially. The FL is located in the incomplete confluence of the union of the body and the lingular process of the greater sphenoid wing anteriorly, the clivus of the occipital bone medially and the petrous apex posteriorly and covered with the fibrocartilaginous tissue that separates the ET from the ICA [23].

b. The internal opening of the CC is located near the FL for the passage of the ICA, which is freed at the petrous apex into the cavernous sinus (**Figure 2**). It is localized medial to the ET, below the greater superficial petrosal nerve (GSPN), a branch of the FN and the trigeminal ganglion [1, 3, 4]. The petrous segment of the ICA within the CC has four anatomic parts, called vertical, posterior genu, horizontal, and anterior genu. During endoscopic endonasal surgery, the junctional part of the ET at the sphenoid spine and FS is crucial landmark to identify and protect the petrous segment of the ICA [13]. The anatomical and surgical relationships between the ET and the petrous segment of the ICA are as follows:

The first curve, posterior genu is located at the level of the bulging basal turn of the cochlea within the bend of the CC. Laterally, the bony part of the ET and the tendon of the tensor tympani muscle; posterolaterally, the promontory and posterosuperiorly, geniculate ganglion are paramount landmarks for the posterior genu of the ICA. The V3 lying anteromedially to the FS and the parapharyngeal segment of the ICA, which passes posteroinferiorly to the sphenoid spine, are critical landmarks. Posterolaterally, the petroclival fissure cartilage is an important landmark to separate the pharyngobasilar fascia from the anterior genu of ICA.

The second turn of the ICA, anterior genu, above the fibrous tissue of the FL is in close proximity to the lacerum segment of the cartilaginous ET laterally and continues as the paraclival ICA in the carotid groove. During the endoscopic approach, the Vidian artery and nerve (VN) are critical landmarks for the second curve of the ICA.

For safe manipulation of the horizontal part of the ICA, the GSPN can be used as surgical landmark. Above the anterolateral margin of the FL the union of the GSPN and the deep petrosal branch of the carotid neural plexus forms the VN which is located anteroinferiorly and lateral to the second turn of the ICA. Malignancies that involve the petrous apex or the carotid artery require the extended endoscopic endonasl approach (EEA). During this procedure, the medial and lateral optico–carotid recesses in the cavernous sinus and the vidian canal (VC) are vital surgical landmarks, which allow to identify the position of the ICA for safe surgical resection near the ICA [13].

c. At the apex above the CC, a shallow fossa called trigeminal impression (**Figure 2**) is located for the lodgement of the sensory ganglion of the TN (semilunar ganglion or Gasser's ganglion) that is covered by a pouch-shaped dura mater called Meckel's cave [3]. Vascular compression and arachnoid adherence of the TN branches result in trigeminal neuralgia. During endoscopic vascular decompression and Meckel's cave approaches, the VC, the bone between V2 and the VC and the pneumatization of the sphenoid sinus form a safe route to access and to decompress Gasser's ganglion with branches, the cranial nerves (III, IV, VI), and the petrous ICA [13, 23].

d. Behind the trigeminal impression, the roof of the IAM is indicated as a shallow fossa, then it continues with the AE, which is a surgical landmark for the middle fossa approach and located at the junction of the posterior third and the anterior two-thirds of the petrous portion (**Figure 2**). It is a valuable guide to signify the SSC and the roof of the vestibule up to 93% of the temporal bones [19, 22].

e. The TT is a thin bony layer covering all of the anterior surface (**Figure 2**). It forms the roof of the mucosal line including from behind to forward the MA, tympanic cavity and ET which are lined with mucosa. Also, its lateral edge turns downward to subdivide the squamo-tympanic fissure into two parts [1, 3].

f. On the TT, a bony roof of the geniculate ganglion, there are two foramina, which continue as a small groove adjoining anteromedially; the medial one starts from the hiatus of the facial canal and lodges the GSPN, a branch of the FN and the petrosal branch of the MMA, whereas the lateral one lodges the lesser superficial petrosal nerve, a branch of GPN (**Figure 2**) [3, 9, 16, 22].

Kaen et al. described the "VELPPHA" area indicating the posterior limit of the transpterygoid EEA. It is composed of the VC (V), the ET (E), the FL (L), the petroclival fissure (P), the pharyngobasilar fascia (PHA), and multiple cartilaginous fibers between them. The posterior opening of the VC, the posterior limit of surgical corridor in the transpterygoid approach, is located above the ET and below the petrous ICA. Behind the posterior margin of the medial pterygoid process, the superomedial border of the ET attaches to the cartilaginous fibers of the FL. The petroclival fissure is situated between the lateral border of the clivus (occipital bone) and the petrous part of the temporal bone and lodges the IPS. The horizontal segment of the petrous ICA turns upward at the medial border of the petrous apex to form the anterior genu of the ICA, and then it continues as the lacerum segment, second vertical segment of the ICA. So, the VC-ET junction is a safe and critical landmark for efficient localization of the lacerum segment of the ICA, as part of the transpterygoid extension of EEA [24].

Tayebi Meybodi et al. described the pterygoclival ligament as a thickened extension of the pharyngobasilar fascia from the pterygoid process to the anteromedial aspect of the lacerum segment of the ICA and reported that the course of the pterygoclival ligament consistently refers to the anteromedial aspect of the lacerum ICA. So, they suggested that the pterygoclival ligament can be used as a safe landmark in case of tumor invasion of the VN, and drilling along the medial aspect of this ligament is more reliable way compared with the VN to avoid the ICA injury during extended EEA. Also, they remarked that this ligament may localize in a venous compartment, which is in contact with the cavernous sinus superiorly and the pterygoid venous plexus posteroinferiorly [25].

2.4.3 Surgical landmarks on the posterior surface of the petrous portion

The posterior surface, anterior wall of the posterior cranial fossa, is encircled by a venous triangle that is formed by the grooves for SS posteriorly and SPS at the petrous ridge and IPS at the junction of the pars lateralis of the occipital bone and the temporal bone anteroinferiorly. The SS drains into the bulb of the IJV, which exists from the JF together with the cranial nerves (IX-XI) [1, 6, 9].

a. The IAM is a short canal, about 1 cm long, and has a large orifice, which allows passage of the vestibulocochlear nerve below the FN, the superficial petrosal artery (a branch of the MMA) and the labyrinthine artery (branch of the basilar artery). The bottom (fundus) of the IAM is subdivided into unequal superior and inferior portions by a transverse falciform crest, and into the anterior and posterior portions by a vertical segment, Bill's bar, respectively (**Figure 3**) [2, 15]. The localization of the nerves within the IAM is determined by a triangular shaped Bill's bar as follows; posteriorly the superior and inferior vestibular nerves, anteroinferiorly the cochlear nerve, anterosuperiorly the FN and nervus intermedius pass through the foramina of the fundus (**Figure 3**) Mortazavi [1, 4, 6].

b. The aqueductus vestibuli is a bony canal which contains the saccus and ductus endolymphaticus. Its opening is an oblique slit behind the IAM (**Figure 3**). The endolymphatic sac is located at the lateral part of the posterior surface medial to the posterior SSC [2, 18].

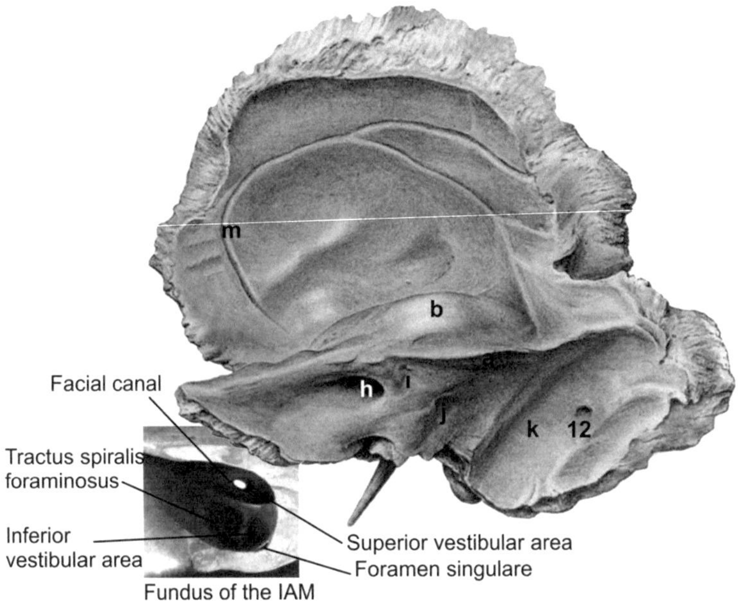

Figure 3.
The surface landmarks on the posterior surface of the petrous portion: a, petrous ridge; b, arcuate eminence; h, internal acoustic meatus; i, subarcuate fossa; j, aqueductus vestibuli; k, sigmoid sinus sulcus; m, sulcus of the middle meningeal artery; 12, mastoid foramen.

c. The subarcuate fossa is an indistinct depression (large in new born) located behind the IAM (**Figure 3**) and transmits a small vein and the subarcuate artery, which is a branch of the meatal segment of the anterior inferior cerebellar artery [4, 5, 9, 14].

2.4.4 Surgical landmarks on the inferior surface of the petrous portion

The inferior surface articulates with the basilar part of occipital bone medially, and the greater wing of the sphenoid bone anteriorly and forms an irregular external surface of the base of the skull. Below the apex, there is a quadrilateral area that serves as an attachment for the levator veli palatini muscle. The lateral part of this area merges with the posterior margin of the greater wing of sphenoid to form the sulcus tuba in front of the cartilaginous portion of the auditory tube [4, 5, 21]. It presents some anatomical landmarks as follows:

1. The external opening of the CC, which shows an inverted L-shape course, forms the entrance for the ICA, which is surrounded by a plexus of sympathetic nerves (**Figure 4**). The anterior margin of the horizontal segment of the CC is separated from the musculotubal canal by a thin layer of bone laterally [1, 5, 18].

2. The jugular fossa is a deep dome-shaped depression at the lateral wall of the JF and located behind the CC and below the floor of the tympanic cavity. It houses the superior bulb of the IJV and the mastoid canaliculus (**Figure 4**) for the entry of the Arnold's nerve, which provides sensory innervation of the EAC and auricle [9, 15]. The jugular spine in the jugular notch of the occipital bone divides the JF into the pars nervosa (anterior) and pars venosa (posterior) [4, 5, 9]. Normally, the jugular bulb is located between the IJV and the

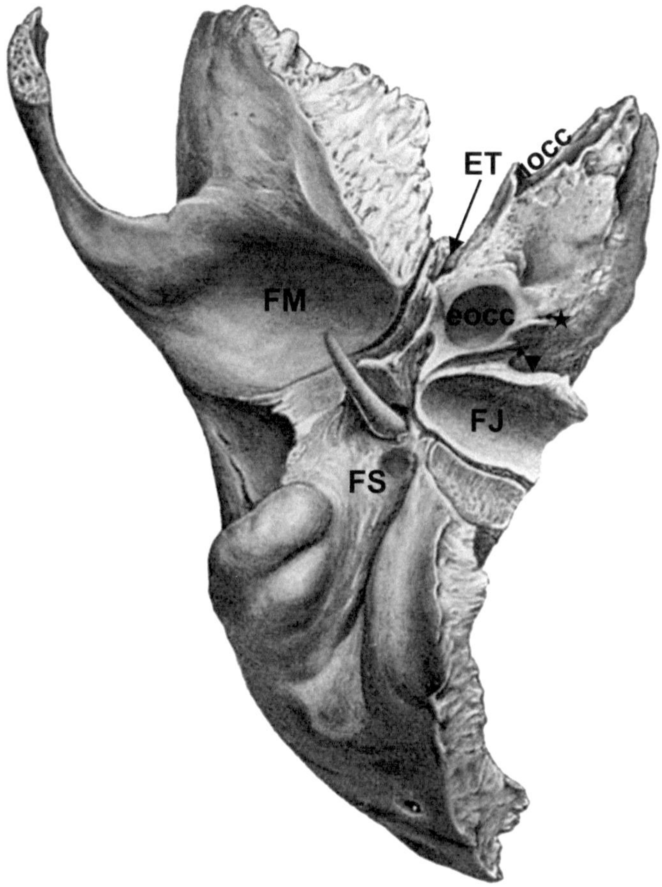

Figure 4.
The surface landmarks on the inferior surface of the petrous portion: FM, fossa mandibularis; FS, foramen stylomastoideum; FJ, fossa jugularis; ET, eustachian tube; eocc, external opening of carotid canal; iocc, internal opening of carotid canal; star: inferior tympanic canaliculus; arrowhead: cochlear aqueduct.

horizontal course of the SS. Abnormalities of it (80% below the FN in the mastoid cavity) result in dehiscence of the adjacent structures such as: the mediolateral enlargement of the JB results in the vestibular aqueduct, PSC, and IAC dehiscence, whereas the anteroposterior enlargement of the JB may cause the FN dehiscence. Abnormal high riding JB shows both mediolateral and anteroposterior enlargement and results in dehiscence of the FN [26].

3. Between the jugular fossa and the CC, the inferior ganglion of the GPN is localized in a triangular depression, whereas the inferior tympanic canaliculus penetrates into wedge-shaped bony ridge and transmits the tympanic branch of the GPN and inferior tympanic artery. At the apex of this triangular depression, there is an external opening of the cochlear aqueduct (**Figure 4**), which connects the perilymphatic space to the subarachnoid space and transmits the cochlear vein [1, 5, 14].

4. Behind the CC the vaginal process which is the extension of the sharp lower border of the tympanic plate wraps the root of the styloid process (**Figure 4**). The lower border of that extension serves an attachment for the deep layer of parotid fascia [1, 3, 5, 6].

2.4.5 Internal anatomy and ossification of the petrous portion

Internal structures in the petrous portion contain the ME and inner ear. The ME contains an air-filled tympanic cavity and the ossicular chain which is composed of the malleus, incus, and stapes [14]. The walls of the ME:

1. Lateral wall contains the tympanic membrane and the scutum pointed infero-medially from the squamous portion. The tympanic membrane has two parts; pars flaccida is located in a fibrocartilaginous ring called the tympanic sulcus and susceptible to perforations and pars tensa is situated in the notch of Rivinus above the lateral process of the malleus. At the medial surface of the membrane a depression called umbo is formed by attachment of the manubrium of the malleus.

2. Medial wall consists of the cochlear promontory, the FC, the oval and round windows. It is divided into three part by the bony ridges: the ponticulus superiorly and the subiculum inferiorly. The oval window (vestibular window) is located above the ponticulus whereas the round window (cochlear window) is below the subiculum, and the tympanic sinus between them is located medial to the FC. The vestibular window is closed by the base of the stapes. The facial recess lies below the lateral SSC and superolateral to the oval window.

3. Superior wall, the TT, which forms the roof of the ME.

4. Inferior wall is a bony roof of the IJV.

5. Anterior wall includes the anterior epitympanic recess superiorly, below it the tensor tympani muscle lies posteriorly and attaches to the neck of the malleus after turning laterally. The orifice of the ET and below it the CC is located inferiorly.

6. Posterior wall consists of the pyramidal eminence, epitympanum, and facial recess. The stapedius muscle passes through the pyramidal eminence and inserts to the head of the stapes [2, 5, 7, 14, 18].

The tympanic cavity is lined with the mucous membrane that extending into the MA posteriorly and the ET anteriorly. This cavity consists of three parts changing according to the level of the tympanic membrane; the epitympanum (superior to the level of the tympanic membrane), mesotympanum (at the level of the tympanic membrane), and hypotympanum (inferior to the level of the tympanic membrane). The hypotympanum has the orifice of the ET. At the lateral part of the epitympanum below the lateral malleal ligament there is the Prussak space which is bounded by the neck of the malleus medially and the pars flaccida and scutum laterally [2, 3, 5, 14].

Inner ear is comprised of the otic capsule (osseous labyrinth), which surrounds the membranous labyrinth and is divided into three parts from anterior to posterior including the cochlea, vestibule, and three SCs [14]. Cochlea is the spiral shaped bony labyrinth of the inner ear that looks like a snail shell making 2¾ turns about the modiolus and consists of the vestibular and the tympanic and the cochlear ducts, which are formed by an inner membranous partition. The vestibular duct (scala vestibuli) locates at the superior part of the cochlear canal and contains perilymph (rich in sodium ions) and is limited by the oval window, and is separated from the cochlear duct by Reissner's membrane. The cochlear duct (scala media) locates at the middle part of the cochlear canal and contains endolymph (rich in potassium ions) and is separated from the tympanic duct by the basilar membrane, which has the Organ of Corti including the sensory hair cells. The stereocilia of these cells perceives the potential difference between the perilymph and the endolymph and converts that motion to electrical signals and finally hearing occurs. The tympanic duct (scala tympani) locates at the inferior part of the cochlear canal and contains perilymph as the vestibular duct and is limited by the round window [3, 5, 14, 15]. Vestibule contains the utricle and saccule. SSCs containing three semicircular ducts organized like three flower leafs that join the vestibule. They are located perpendicular to each other; the superior corresponds to the AE, the posterior is parallel to the posterior surface of the pyramid, and the lateral is perpendicular the mucosal plane and angled at 30°from the transverse plane [3, 15].

The FN passes through the anterosuperior part of the IAM and enters the fallopian canal (FC). It contains motor, sensory, and parasympathetic fibers and has six segments as follows:

1. Cisternal segment lies from the brain stem to the IAM. This part runs together with the cisternal part of vestibulocochlear nerve in same pia mater coverage.

2. Meatal segment is the smallest part of the FC and contains Bill's bar as an important landmark.

3. Petrous (labyrinthine) segment forms first genu (geniculate ganglion) above the cochlea at the lateral wall of the ME and gives a branch named as GSPN. Then, it enters the tympanic cavity and forms an angle ranging from 19 to 107° with tympanic segment of the FC [7, 20]. Because of this segment is the narrowest part and lack of arterial anastomoses, it is susceptible to embolic attacks and vascular compression.

4. Tympanic segment (first part) starts from first genu and turns backwards to lie in a thin-walled bony canal that runs evenly between the lateral SSC superiorly and the oval window inferiorly and medial to the incus. A dehiscence of the bony canal is more common at this segment in average 41–75%.

5. Pyramidal segment (second part of the tympanic segment) forms second genu at the posterior wall of the ME above the pyramidal process. It forms an angle ranging from 95 to 125° with mastoid segment of the FC [7, 20].

6. In the mastoid or vertical segment, the FN gives the acoustic branch for the stapedius muscle, the chorda tympani, and sensitive branch for the auricular region. This segment is located 5.50 mm anteromedially to the SS and extends from the level of the LSC to the digastric ridge (~3.8 mm). Then it exits the temporal bone at the SMF and enters the parotid gland [14, 27].

According to the classical description, the FC has four segments: labyrinthine, tympanic, pyramidal, and mastoid, but the meatal segment is important from an anatomical and surgical perspective. The stylomastoid artery, a branch of the posterior auricular or the occipital arteries, supplies the inferior parts of the FC up to the second genu and anastomoses directly with the petrosal branch of the MMA, which supplies the geniculate ganglion. The FC pathologies are composed of agenesis, aplasia, narrowing, and osteopetrosis of the canal, which result in complete or incomplete facial paralysis. Bell's palsy depending on the activation of a dormant herpes virus, is responsible for 50% of peripheral FN palsies. The FC dehiscence can be congenital or secondary to the surgical intervention or pathology of adjacent structures and results in cerebrospinal fluid (CSF) otorrhea. Several surgical approaches, including the translabyrinthine, transcochlear and retrosigmoid, are used to treat the FC pathologies [27].

Ossification of the petrous portion begins from the 14 centers that fuse to form otic capsule and is completed at birth. The petrous portion develops from the cartilaginous differentiation of the mesenchyme by endochondral ossification at the 16th week of gestation. The cementum layer in teeth roots and petrous portion of the temporal bone contain the optimal endogenous DNA substrate which can provide information to specify the geographic location for genomic analyses [28]. Damgaard et al. reported that the prevalence of the endogenous DNA contents in nonpetrous bones and teeth is ranged from 0.3 to 20.7%, while the levels for petrous bones ranges between 37.4 and 85.4% [29]. Due to the high density and resistance to harsher climatic conditions of the petrous bone, the otic capsule of the petrous bone preserves DNA substrate extremely well and has much higher endogenous DNA level than the teeth by 5.2-fold on average. So, it is currently acknowledged as the optimal substrates for ancient genomic research [28, 29].

2.4.6 Triangles on the anterior and posterior surfaces of the petrous portion

Kawase's triangle: Borghei-Razavi et al. evaluated the safety of this posteromedial middle fossa triangle for removal of the tumors locating or spreading into the cerebellopontine angle and petroclival area. Kawase's triangle was identified

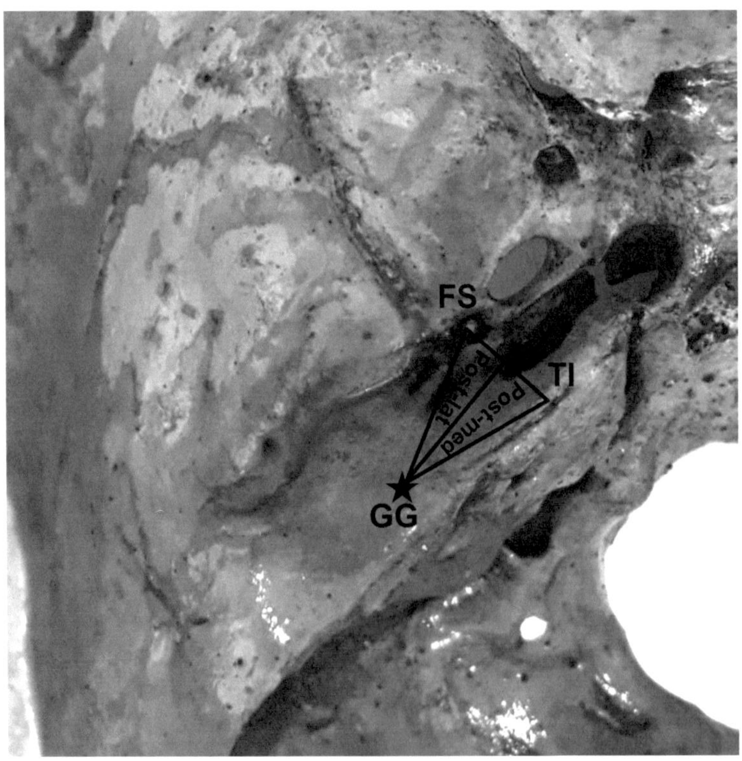

Figure 5.
The surgical triangles on the anterior surface: Kawase's triangle: Post-med (posteromedial triangle) and Glasscock's triangle: post-lat (posterolateral triangle). FS, foramen spinosum; GG, geniculate ganglion; TI, trigeminal impression.

between the GSPN laterally, the geniculate ganglion at the AE posteriorly, and ganglion gasserian at the trigeminal impression anteriorly. During anterior petrosectomy for accessing the posterior cranial fossa via middle fossa, the GSPN forms the lateral border of the surgical approach (**Figure 5**) [30].

Glasscock's triangle, or the posterolateral middle fossa triangle, is identified between the TN (V3), the geniculate ganglion at the AE and FS (**Figure 5**). The margins of this triangle are formed by a line between where the GSPN crosses under V3 and the FS medially, a line between the FS and geniculate ganglion laterally, and GSPN describing the base [3, 5, 16].

Rhomboid area (Kawase triangle+postmeatal area) is situated between the GPN, petrous ridge, AE, and the posterior border of the V3. A large tumor located in the midline skull base or spreading into the infratemporal and petroclival region even the cavernous sinus can be removed by extended EEA through V2-V3 corridor to avoid complications including ICA injury, IPS bleeding, TN injury and CSF leak [31].

Trautmann's triangle is bounded by the SPS superiorly, SS posteriorly, and solid angle which is formed by three SCs anteriorly (**Figure 6**). In this triangle, the retrolabyrinthine tract from the MA, the endolymphatic sac, and the vestibular aqueduct are located [5, 9].

Donaldson's line is a surgical line that is parallel to the LSC whereas it is vertical to the posterior SSC and divide it into superior and inferior portions. Below this line medial to the labyrinth the endolymphatic sac is situated. Citelli's angle (sinodural angle); is bounded by the middle fossa dura plate (SPS) superiorly, posterior fossa dura plate (bony plate covering the MA) anteriorly and the SS posteriorly (**Figure 6**). During mastoidectomy the air cells in this triangle should be removed [1, 5, 6].

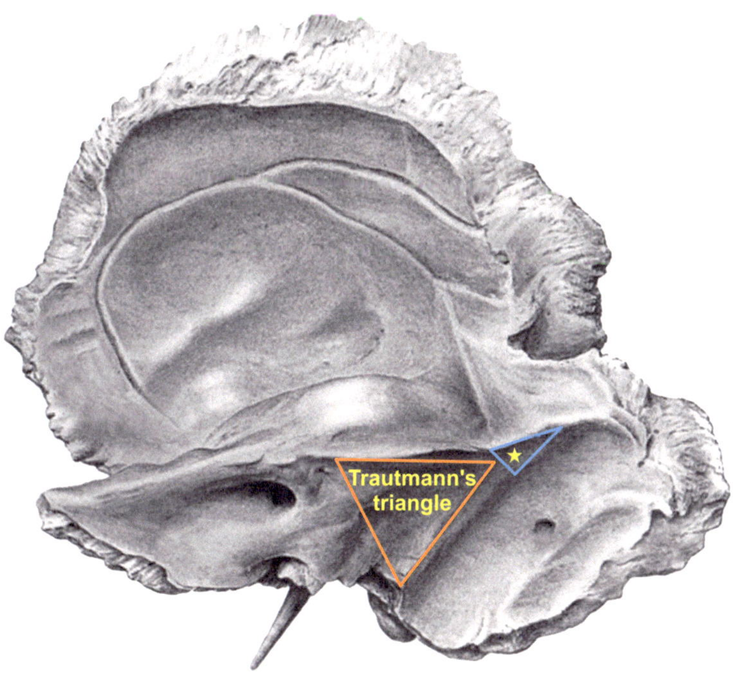

Figure 6.
The surgical triangles on the posterior surface: Trautmann's triangle margins are formed between the superior petrosal sinus superiorly, the sigmoid sinus posteriorly, and the semicircular canals antero-inferiorly. Star: Citelli's angle (sinodural angle) is formed between the dural plates of the middle fossa superiorly, the posterior fossa anteriorly and the sigmoid sinus posteriorly.

3. Segmental anatomy of the petrous portion

In clinical applications, for fully understanding of the tridimensional architecture of the petrous portion, a reference lines and angles can be defined on the anterior and posterior surfaces from a superior view.

Peris-Celda et al. reported that the EAM and the IAM are located in the same coronal plane on the anterior surface forming surgical triangle [9]. Tawfik-Helika et al. separated the pyramid into four compartments and described two segmentation method to provide better understanding of the distributions of these compartments. They identified four compartments based on their connections: mucosal, cutaneous, neural, and vascular [3, 21].

The mucosal compartment consists of an air filled and mucosa lined cavities from anterior to posterior: the ET, ME, and the MA (**Figure 7**). The mucosal line in an oblique anteromedial direction extends along these structures and is used for segmental description of this pyramid, and all major anatomical landmarks can be identified relative to this axis for surgical approaches [3, 9, 21].

Extending the mucosal line posteriorly, the MA is separated into medial and lateral parts, whereas anteriorly, the bony portion of the ET is localized at the junction of the petrous and squamous parts and the cartilaginous part opens into the pharynx anteriorly. Medially the line passing through the sulcus of the GSPN and laterally a straight line lying between the foramen ovale and FS are parallel to this line (**Figure 7**) [3, 9, 21].

The cutaneous compartment is composed of the EAM, which is covered by the skin and separated from the ME by the tympanic membrane medially.

The neural compartment is composed of the otic capsule, which is located medial to ME and the mucosal line. In this bony container, the cochlea, vestibule, and SCs are located from anterior to posterior around the fundus of the IAM (**Figure 7**).

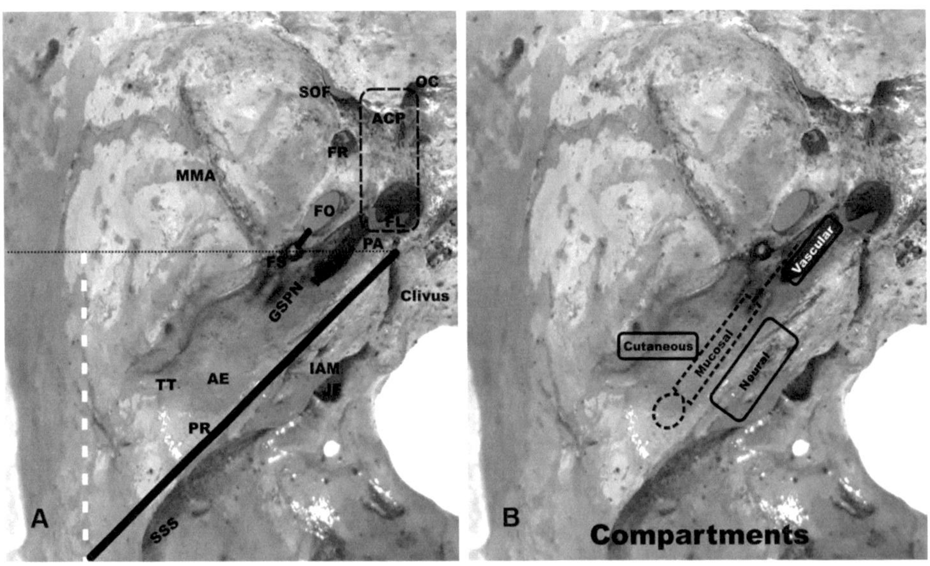

Figure 7.
(A) The margins of the anterior surface of the left petrous portion from a superior view are shown posteriorly by a (thick black) line along the PR, petrous ridge; anteriorly by a (dashed black) line lying from the preauricular burrhole to PA, petrous apex and passing through the FS, foramen spinosum; and laterally by a (dashed white) line along the petro-squamous suture. OC, optic canal; ACP, anterior clinoid process; FL, foramen lacerum; SOF, superior orbital fissure; FR, foramen rotundum; FO, foramen ovale; MMA, middle meningeal artery; IOCC, internal opening of carotid canal; GSPN, greater petrosal nerve; AE, arcuate eminence; TT, tegmen tympani; JF, jugular foramen; IAM, internal acoustic meatus; SSS, sulcus sigmoid sinus. (B) The segmentation of the left petrous pyramid into four compartments including mucosal, cutaneous, neural, and vascular is shown on the left petrous portion.

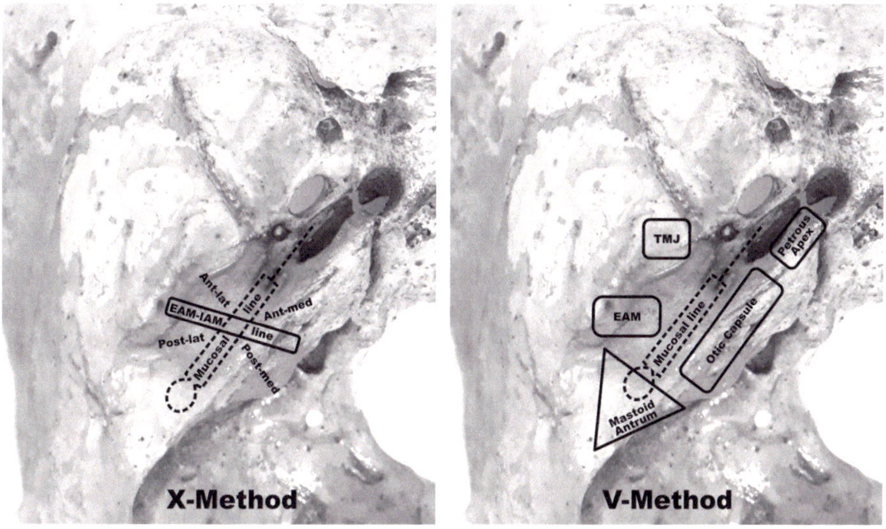

Figure 8.
Schematic representations of the segmentation of the left petrous portion by using X and V methods.

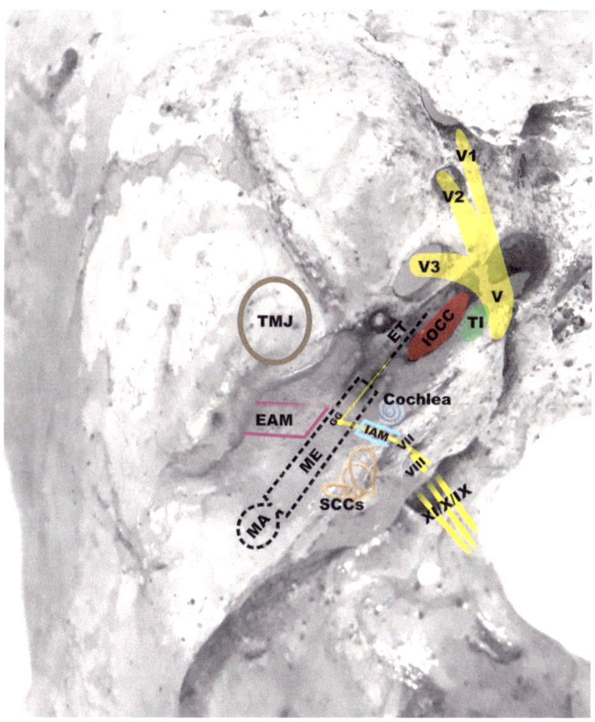

Figure 9.
Schematic representation of the external and internal landmarks on the left petrous portion. V, trigeminal nerve and branches (V1, V2, V3); TI, trigeminal impression; IOCC, internal opening of carotid canal; ET, Eustachian tube; GG, geniculate ganglion; ME, middle ear; MA; mastoid antrum; EAM, external acoustic meatus; TMJ, temporomandibular joint; SCCs, semicircular canals; IAM, internal acoustic meatus; VII, facial nerve; VIII, vestibulocochlear nerve; IX, glossopharyngeal nerve; X, vagus nerve; XI, accessory nerve.

The vascular compartment is composed of the ICA. The axis passing through the horizontal part of the CC is parallel and medial to the mucosal line (**Figure 7**) [3]. Moreover, Tawfik-Helika et al. described X and V segmentation methods to advance and enhance education of the compartments.

The X method divides the petrous pyramid into four spaces by using two reference lines intersecting with each other at the ME; the mucosal line and the EAM-IAM line form the X letter (**Figures 8** and **9**). These four spaces around the ME and the contents in it are as follows:

The anteromedial space—the cochlea and the petrous apex including the ICA

The anterolateral space—the roof of the TMJ

The posterolateral space—the lateral part of the MA

The posteromedial space—the posterior labyrinth and the medial part of the MA

The V method arranges five segments around the mucosal line (**Figures 8** and **9**)

These five segments and the contents in it are as follows:

The petrous apex segment—the ICA medial to the ET

The otic capsule segment—the IAM, cochlea, vestibule and SCs

The mastoid segment—the angle around the MA

The EAM segment—the lateral part of the ME

The TMJ segment—the roof of the TMJ lateral to the ET [3].

4. Conclusions

Detailed description of the temporal anatomy pointing to relationships between internal and external landmarks and a holistic approach including X an V segmentation methods that break down the petrous pyramid into spaces and compartments can provide an easy way to understand and to use surgical applications. The compartmental approach can be helpful in the fields of education and radiological applications as well as surgery.

Author details

Gülay Açar and Aynur Emine Çiçekcibaşı*

Department of Anatomy, Meram Faculty of Medicine, Necmettin Erbakan University, Konya, Turkey

*Address all correspondence to: aynurcicekcibasi@yahoo.com.tr

References

[1] Mansour S, Magnan J, Haidar H, Nicolas KSL. Comprehensive and Clinical Anatomy of the Middle Ear. 1st ed. Heidelberg: Springer-Verlag; 2013

[2] Juliano AF, Ginat DT, Moonis G. Imaging review of the temporal bone: Part I. Anatomy and inflammatory and neoplastic processes. Radiology. 2013;**269**(1):17-33

[3] Tawfik-Helika M, Mertens P, Ribas G, Cusimano MD, Catala M, Kirollos R, et al. Understanding anatomy of the petrous pyramid-a new compartmental approach. World Neurosurgery. 2019;**124**:e65-e80

[4] Powell KA, Kashikar T, Hittle B, Stredney D, Kerwin T, Wiet GJ. Atlas-based segmentation of temporal bone surface structures. International Journal of Computer Assisted Radiology and Surgery. 2019;**14**(8):1267-1273

[5] Gray SS. Gray's Anatomy: The Anatomical Basis of Clinical Practice. Philadelphia: Elsevier; 2016

[6] Belsare GS. Step by Step Temporal Bone Dissection. New Delhi, India: Jaypee Brothers Medical Publishers; 2014

[7] Alhussaini MA, Mattingly JK, Cass SP. Anatomical relationship of the middle cranial fossa dura to surface landmarks of the temporal bone. Otology & Neurotology. 2017;**38**(9):1351-1354. DOI: 10.1097/MAO.0000000000001532

[8] Bender ME, Lipin RB, Goudy SL. Development of the pediatric temporomandibular joint. Oral and Maxillofacial Surgery Clinics of North America. 2018;**30**(1):1-9. DOI: 10.1016/j.coms.2017.09.002

[9] Peris-Celda M, Perry A, Carlstrom LP, Graffeo CS, Driscoll CLW, Link MJ. Key anatomical landmarks for middle fossa surgery: A surgical anatomy study. Journal of Neurosurgery. 2018;**131**:1561-1570. DOI: 10.3171/2018.5.JNS1841

[10] Lee HJ, Choi YJ, Lee KW, Kim HJ. Positional patterns among the auriculotemporal nerve, superficial temporal artery, and superficial temporal vein for use in decompression treatments for migraine. Scientific Reports. 2018;**8**(1):16539. DOI: 10.1038/s41598-018-34765-1

[11] Todd NW. Helpful and unhelpful parts of the superior petrosal triangle. Otolaryngology and Head and Neck Surgery. 2006;**134**(6):966-969

[12] Baur DA, Beushausen M, Leech B, Quereshy F, Fitzgerald N. Anatomic study of the distance between the articular eminence and foramen spinosum and foramen spinosum and petrotympanic fissure. Journal of Oral and Maxillofacial Surgery. 2014;**72**(6):1125-1129. DOI: 10.1016/j.joms.2013.12.030

[13] Oyama K, Tahara S, Hirohata T, Ishii Y, Prevedello DM, Carrau RL, et al. Surgical anatomy for the endoscopic endonasal approach to the ventrolateral skull base. Neurologia Medico-Chirurgica (Tokyo). 2017;**57**(10):534-541

[14] Juliano AF. Cross sectional imaging of the ear and temporal bone. Head and Neck Pathology. 2018;**12**(3):302-320

[15] Benson JC, Eckel L, Guerin J, Silvera VM, Diehn F, Passe T, et al. Review of temporal bone microanatomy: Aqueducts, canals, clefts and nerves. Clinical Neuroradiology. 2019;**30**(2):209-219. DOI: 10.1007/s00062-019-00864-3

[16] Altieri R, Sameshima T, Pacca P, Crobeddu E, Garbossa D, Ducati A, et al.

Detailed anatomy knowledge: First step to approach petroclival meningiomas through the petrous apex. Anatomy lab experience and surgical series. Neurosurgical Review. 2017;**40**(2):231-239

[17] Przewozny TT, Kosinski A, Markiet K, Sierszen W, Kuczkowski J, Kurylowicz J, et al. Körner's septum (petrosquamosal lamina): The anatomical variant or clinical problem? Folia Morphologica. 2020;**79**(2): 205-210. DOI: 10.5603/FM.a2019.0079

[18] Isaacson B. Anatomy and surgical approach of the ear and temporal bone. Head and Neck Pathology. 2018;**12**(3):321-327

[19] Deniz Y, Geduk G, Zengin AZ. Examination of foramen tympanicum: An anatomical study using cone-beam computed tomography. Folia Morphologica. 2018;**77**(2):335-339

[20] Mittal S, Singal S, Mittal A, Singal R, Jindal G. Identification of foramen of Huschke with reversible herniation of temporomandibular joint soft tissue into the external auditory canal on multidetector computed tomography. Proceedings (Baylor University Medical Center). 2017;**30**(1):92-93. DOI: 10.1080/08998280.2017.11929544

[21] Pellet W, Cannoni M, Pech A. Otoneurosurgery. Berlin: Springer; 2012

[22] Singh A, Kumar R, Irugu DVK, Kumar R, Sagar P. Morphometric analysis of arcuate eminence: A distinctive landmark for middle cranial fossa approach. Journal of Cranio-Maxillo-Facial Surgery. 2018;**46**(10):1703-1706. DOI: 10.1371/journal.pone.0129102

[23] Brown EC, Lucke-Wold B, Cetas JS, Dogan A, Gupta S, Hullar TE, et al. Surgical parameters for minimally invasive trans–eustachian tube csf leak repair: A cadaveric study and literature review. World Neurosurgery. 2019;**122**:e121-e129. DOI: 10.1016/j.wneu.2018.09.123

[24] Kaen A, Ruiz-Valdepeñas EC, Di Somma A, Esteban F, Rivas JM, Fernandez JA. Refining the anatomic boundaries of the endoscopic endonasal transpterygoid approach: The "VELPPHA area" concept. Journal of Neurosurgery. 2018;**131**(3):911-919. DOI: 10.3171/2018.4.JNS173070

[25] Tayebi Meybodi AS, Little A, Vigo V, Benet A, Kakaizada ST, Lawton M. The pterygoclival ligament: A novel landmark for localization of the internal carotid artery during the endoscopic endonasal approach. Journal of Neurosurgery. 2018;**18**:1-11. DOI: 10.3171/2017.12.JNS172435

[26] Cömert E, Kiliç C, Cömert A. Jugular bulb anatomy for lateral skull base approaches. The Journal of Craniofacial Surgery. 2018;**29**(7):1969-1972. DOI: 10.1097/SCS.0000000000004637

[27] Mortazavi MM, Latif B, Verma K, Adeeb N, Deep A, Griessenauer CJ, et al. The Fallopian Canal: A comprehensive review and proposal of a new classification. Child's Nervous System. 2014;**30**(3):387-395. DOI: 10.1007/s00381-013-2332-0

[28] Hansen HB, Damgaard PB, Margaryan A, Stenderup J, Lynnerup N, Willerslev E, et al. Comparing ancient DNA preservation in petrous bone and tooth cementum. PLoS One. 2017;**12**(1):e0170940

[29] Damgaard PB, Margaryan A, Schroeder H, Orlando L, Willerslev E, Allentoft ME. Improving access to endogenous DNA in ancient bones and teeth. Scientific Reports. 2015;**5**:11184. DOI: 10.1038/srep11184

[30] Borghei-Razavi H, Tomio R, Fereshtehnejad SM, Shibao S, Schick U, Toda M, et al. Anterior petrosal approach: The safety of kawase triangle as an anatomical landmark for anterior petrosectomy in petroclival meningiomas. Clinical Neurology and Neurosurgery. 2015;**139**:282-287. DOI: 10.1016/j.clineuro.2015.10.032

[31] Watanabe K, Zomorodi AR, Labidi M, Satoh S, Froelich S, Fukushima T. Visualization of dark side of skull base with surgical navigation and endoscopic assistance: Extended petrous rhomboid and rhomboid with maxillary nerve-mandibular nerve vidian corridor. World Neurosurgery. 2019;**129**:e134-e145. DOI: 10.1016/j.wneu.2019.05.062

Chapter 2

Surgical Anatomy of the Tonsils

Gülay Açar

Abstract

The tonsils represent a circular band of mucosa associated with lymphoid tissues, Waldeyer's ring, which is located at the entrance of the upper aerodigestive tract, with a significant role in the immune defense system. Waldeyer's ring is composed of the pharyngeal, tubal, palatine, and lingual tonsils acting as secondary lymphoid tissues. Particularly, the palatine tonsils are the largest of the tonsils with deep branching crypts and contain B and T lymphocytes and M cell which plays a role in the uptake and transport of antigens. Because of the tonsil enlargement during childhood, upper airway obstruction and obstructive sleep apnea syndrome are mostly seen. Knowledge of the surgical anatomy of the tonsils and variations of the neurovascular and muscular structures around it allows optimal choice of surgical technique to avoid iatrogenic complications during tonsillectomy. Recent medical studies reported that a detailed understanding of the anatomic risk factors in upper airway obstruction allows to predict treatment response to surgical intervention. Due to the penetration of benign or malign lesions of the tonsil into the lateral wall of the pharynx, transoral robotic approach to this region is necessary to identify the surgical anatomic landmarks which are required to perform safe and effective surgical intervention.

Keywords: palatine tonsil, parapharyngeal space, surgical anatomy, transoral robotic surgery, Waldeyer's ring

1. Introduction

As part of secondary lymphoid organs, mucosa-associated lymphoid tissue (MALT) is an aggregate of unencapsulated lymphoid tissue that is located diffusely in the mucosa of the aerodigestive tract and consists of the tonsils, vermiform appendix, and Peyer's patch [1]. As part of MALT, the tonsils serve as a protection ring including nasopharynx-associated lymphoid tissue (NALT), which is known as Waldeyer's tonsillar ring, around the entrance of the upper aerodigestive tract to start the initial immunological barrier to infections [1, 2]. This annular-shaped lymphoid ring contains four types of tonsils in a fixed position [3].

1. Pharyngeal (adenoid) tonsil

2. Eustachian tube tonsils (Gerlach's tonsils)

3. Lingual tonsils and lymphoid aggregations close to the epiglottis

4. The palatine (faucial) tonsils

Due to the close proximity of the palatine tonsil with the surrounding spaces including parapharyngeal, retropharyngeal, masticator, and parotid spaces, the tumors and inflammation of the tonsil commonly spread into these spaces and result in secondary lesions [4, 5]. A detailed knowledge of the surgical anatomic landmarks in the tonsillar region and the spaces around it is required for preoperative planning and to prevent iatrogenic complications.

2. Immune function of the tonsils in Waldeyer's ring

The tonsils are lymphoepithelial organs acting as a guardian at the entrance of the upper aerodigestive tract. Lymphoid system, as a component of the immune system, consists of lymph vessels, nodes, and organs that regulate the immune response directly or indirectly. The lymph vessels play a key role in the drainage of interstitial fluid from the tissues to the blood and fat absorption, whereas the lymphoid organs mediate the proliferation and maturation of the cells of the immune system, which protect the body against ingested or inhaled foreign pathogens. The cell groups of the immune system, which is known as the ability to distinguish self from nonself, produce two reactions that are called the innate (natural) and adaptive (acquired) immunity [1, 2]. Initially, lymphocytes and accessory cells are developed and matured to the stage of antigen recognition in primary lymphoid organs including the thymus and bone marrow, and then they are activated and differentiated to effector cells of the immune response by antigen presentation in secondary lymphoid organs. The lymph nodes, the spleen, and mucosa-associated lymphoid tissue are secondary lymphoid organs which allow lymphocytes to become functional to produce a defense mechanism against microorganisms such as viruses, parasites, and bacteria. The structures of MALT have 70% of all the cells of the immune system, and the percentages of the lymphocytes in each of them are variable [1].

3. Anatomical localization of the tonsils in the pharynx

As part of the upper aerodigestive tract, the pharynx is located between the skull base and the inferior border of cricoid cartilage and consists of three portions; the nasopharynx (upper nasal), oropharynx (middle oral), and laryngopharynx (lower laryngeal). It is a musculomembranous tube covered with three external (circular, the superior, middle, and inferior constrictors) and three internal (longitudinal, voluntary) muscles, which play a key role in swallowing, respiration, and phonation [6]. The tonsils are located posterior to the nasal and oral portions of the pharynx to form a circumferential ring, known as the Waldeyer's tonsillar ring, which was first described by German anatomist Heinrich Wilhelm Gottfried von Waldeyer-Hartz [3]. The unpaired nasopharyngeal and lingual tonsils and the paired palatine and tubal tonsils form Waldeyer's lymphoid ring at the opening of the upper aerodigestive tract and are responsible for both innate and adaptive immunological responses which have a crucial role in the defense mechanism of the pharynx (**Figure 1**) [7].

3.1 Nasopharynx

As a part of the upper respiratory system, the nasopharynx is bounded by the choanae anteriorly, the upper surface of the soft palate inferiorly, and the

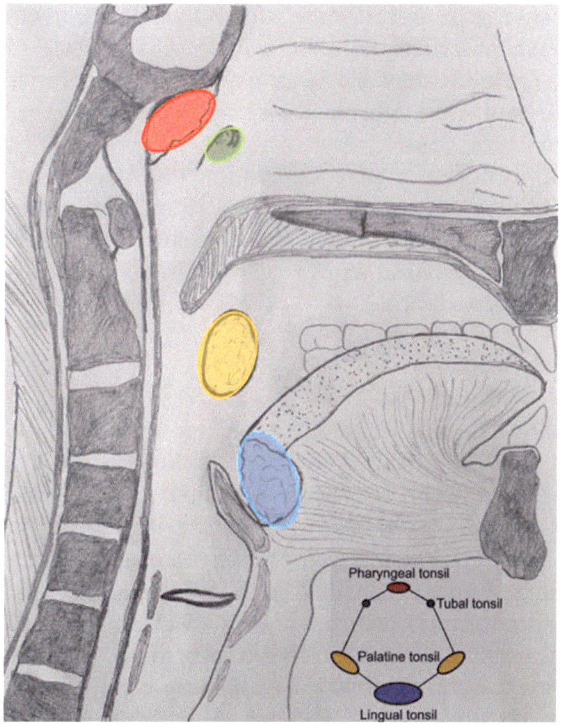

Figure 1.
The localization of the tonsils in Waldeyer's tonsillar ring.

oropharyngeal isthmus (OPI) posterolaterally. The nasopharyngeal and tubal tonsils are located in the posterolateral wall of the nasopharynx [6]. The palatoglossal arch (PGa) and palatopharyngeal arch (PPa) join with each other to form the OPI which allows the communication with the oropharynx. The boundaries of the OPI are formed by the soft palate (velum) anteriorly and the lateral and posterior pharyngeal walls posterolaterally. During swallowing and speaking, the levator veli palatini (LVPm), palatopharyngeus (PPm), superior pharyngeal constrictor (SPCm), salpingopharyngeus (SPm), and the uvula, which are called a velopharyngeal sphincter, play a role in the closure of the OPI. During velopharyngeal function, a transverse mucosal ridge called Passavant's ridge (palatopharyngeal sphincter) runs along the posterior wall of the OPI between the most lateral part (transverse fibers) of the PPm and the most superior part of the SPCm [7, 8].

3.2 Pharyngeal tonsil

Pharyngeal tonsil is the superior-most of the Waldeyer's ring and located above the soft palate in the posterosuperior roof of the nasopharynx as a single median unencapsulated mass with 12–15 shallow, crypt-like invaginations. The pharyngeal bursa, a blind mucosal sac, may be seen in the posterior median wall of the nasopharynx above the SPCm. A median longitudinal groove extends from this sac inferiorly [6]. Anterosuperiorly, the pharyngeal tonsil is usually lined by pseudostratified ciliated columnar epithelium (respiratory epithelium), whereas posteroinferiorly the areas adjacent to the oropharynx is covered by stratified epithelium. These mucosal folds containing numerous lymphoid nodules commonly enlarge and become adenoid which results in respiratory difficulties and nasal obstruction during childhood and often start to involute after 7 years of age or even atrophied in the adult. Chronic inflammation of the pharyngeal tonsil results in hyperplasia and hypertrophy of the lymphoid tissue known as adenoid [7].

The arterial supply of it comes from ascending pharyngeal artery, pharyngeal branch of the maxillary artery, artery of the pterygoid canal, basisphenoid artery, ascending palatine, and tonsillar branch of the facial artery. It has a lymphatic drainage into upper deep cervical within the parapharyngeal space (PPS) and retropharyngeal lymph nodes [7].

3.3 Tubal tonsils

Eustachian tube (ET) tonsils, small aggregates of lymphoid tissue, form the upper lateral aspect of the ring and are located bilaterally around the pharyngeal ostium of the ET (torus tubarius) which is below and in front of the pharyngeal recess (fossa of Rosenmüller) in the posterolateral wall of the nasopharynx [6]. Because of their close relationship to the torus tubarius, they are called tubal or Gerlach's (German anatomist) tonsils. This triangular pharyngeal ostium has three prominences: anterior, posterior, and inferior. The anterior fold continues as a plica salpingopalatina descends into the soft palate. The posterior prominence is conspicuous and formed by the projecting cartilage of the auditory tube, called the torus tubarius, and also lies as plica salpingopharyngeus which is composed of the SPm. The torus tubarius can be used for ET catheterization. On the lower aspect of the ostium, the LVPm insertion forms a slightly rounded prominence [6, 7].

Tubal tonsils are covered by pseudostratified ciliated columnar epithelium with no crypts. They receive arterial supply via the ascending pharyngeal artery. Their lymphatic drainage is the same as the pharyngeal tonsil's [6, 7].

3.4 Oropharynx

The oropharynx extends from the OPI at the level of the soft palate to hyoid bone (C3 vertebra level). Anteriorly, the oropharynx communicates with the oral cavity via isthmus faucium which is limited by the PGa bilaterally, the uvula superiorly, and the posterior one third of the tongue that is in line with the sulcus terminalis inferiorly. According to the oncologic description, the oropharynx consists of four parts: the soft palate, the pharyngeal wall, the base of the tongue, and the palatine tonsillar fossa. So, a thorough understanding of the anatomy of oropharyngeal parts and adjacent structures is paramount in differential diagnosis and surgical interventions. It contains the palatine tonsils laterally and lingual tonsil in the retrolingual region anteriorly [6, 9].

3.5 Lingual tonsil

Lingual tonsils are the inferior-most of the ring and composed of numerous lymphoid nodules in the posterior third of the tongue. The stratified squamous nonkeratinized epithelium covers this lymphoid tissue aggregates forming large, irregular protrusions. Also, they have less branching shallow crypts which are covered by the reticulated epithelium and mucous salivary glands which are drained through several ducts into these crypts which appear after birth [6, 9].

Vascular supply to the lingual tonsils is provided with the dorsal lingual branches of the lingual artery and vein. Efferent lymphatic vessels of the lingual tonsil passing through the pharyngeal wall drain into the deep cervical lymph nodes [6, 7, 9].

3.6 Anatomy of the palatine tonsils

The palatine tonsils are two large, conspicuous almond-shaped mass of the lymphoid tissue forming the lower lateral aspect of the ring and localized in a triangular tonsillar fossa along the anterolateral border of the oropharynx on each side. The dimensions of the tonsils are about 10–15 mm in width and 20–25 mm in length in adults, but increase in children. The surface landmark of the tonsil corresponds to the lower part of masseter muscle in front of the angle of mandible [3, 6, 9]. The palatoglossal (anterior pillar) and palatopharyngeal (posterior pillar) mucosal folds diverge from the soft palate to form the boundaries of the tonsillar fossa, which lodges the palatine tonsils. These mucosal arches consist of the palatoglossal muscle (PGm) anteriorly and the PPm posteriorly. The palatine tonsil has two poles, upper and lower; two borders, anterior and posterior; two surfaces, medial and lateral; three mucosal folds, plica semilunaris, plica triangularis, and plica retrotonsillaris; and two depressions, supratonsillar and anterior tonsillar fossa [3, 6, 7].

3.6.1 Poles

Superiorly, the tonsil is free and expands into the soft palate where both arches join.

Inferiorly, the suspensory ligament, a band of fibrous tissue, connects the lower pole with the posterior one third of the tongue. Most of carcinomas develop in the tonsillolingual sulcus which separates the tonsil from tongue anteroinferiorly [3, 6].

3.6.2 Borders

The tonsillar fossa or sinus is a triangular space between the anterior pillar in front, the posterior pillar behind, and the dorsal surface of the posterior one third of the tongue inferiorly (**Figure 2**). Because the tonsils are positioned in it, its borders also limit the tonsil [7].

The anterior boundary is formed by the PGa which is composed of the PGm. A cylindrical muscle extends from the palatine aponeurosis to the posterolateral surface of the tongue and becomes continuous with the intrinsic transverse muscles [6, 7]. It acts as an antagonist of the LVPm and constricts the OPI during swallowing. All of the muscles of the tongue derive from the occipital myotomes except the PGm which is derivation of the fourth branchial arch. According to the variations of the origin of the PGm, the tongue elevator's function increases or decreases. During lateral pharyngoplasty, the relaxation of the SPCm and PGm is provided by the myotomy of these muscles [3, 10].

The posterior boundary is formed by the PPa including the PPm which originates from the palatine aponeurosis and the median part of soft palate by two heads and consists of muscle bundles medial and lateral to the LVPm. The lateral fibers of the PPm are composed of the longitudinal and transverse parts. The transverse part inserts into the pharyngeal raphe to join with the contralateral side, whereas the longitudinal part joins with the medial fibers at the posterior border of the soft palate and afterward are merged by the SPm [7, 8, 11]. This muscle bundle is observed to course downward along the inner surface of pharyngeal wall and inserts into

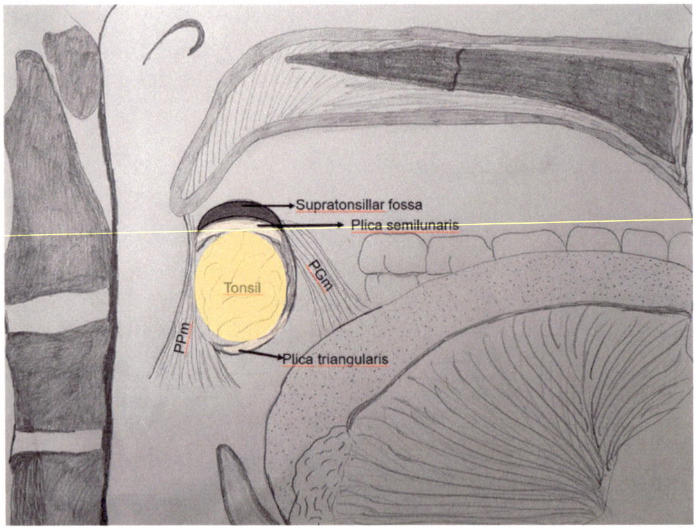

Figure 2.
The mucosal folds and arches of the palatine tonsil.

the palatal tonsil to form the posterior pillar. Also, some of its fibers insert into the posterior border of the thyroid cartilage with the stylopharyngeus muscle (StPm) and into the SPCm [11].

During velopharyngeal closure, the PPm performs various functions such as a sphincter with the SPCm, a puller of the pharyngeal wall medially in collaboration with the SPCm and StPm, and an elevator with the StPm because of the fibers of the PPm running in various directions [8, 11].

3.6.3 Mucosal folds

In the 14th–15th week of gestation, the primitive tonsil and tonsillar fossa develop indirectly from the endoderm part of the second pharyngeal arch. At first, the tonsil has two lobes and a plica intratonsillaris (intratonsillar cleft) between them. This plica later usually disappears, but it may infrequently transform into crypta magna [6, 12]. Because the tonsil does not completely fill this fossa, two small depressions exist at the upper and anteroinferior parts of the tonsillar fossa. They are separated from the tonsil by mucosal folds, known as the plica semilunaris and triangularis, which are remnants of the primitive tonsillar fossa (**Figure 2**) [6, 7].

Superiorly the plica semilunaris originates from the upper aspect of the PGa and extends backward toward the PPa along the upper pole of the tonsil. It encloses a small depression that is known as supratonsillar fossa which separates the tonsil from the uvula [6, 7].

Anteroinferiorly the plica triangularis, an inconstant mucosal fold, arises from the PGa and covers the anteroinferior part of the tonsil. It encloses a smaller fossa that is known as anterior tonsillar fossa, which is then obscured by its walls and forms the imbedded portion of the tonsil [6, 7].

Also, the plica infratonsillaris or retrotonsillaris may extend to the PPa at the posteroinferior part of the tonsil [7]. At first there is no lymphoid tissue in these fossae, but in childhood, they are usually transformed into lymphoid tissues, which are an exclusive hiding place for a constant lithified secretion and foreign bodies, causing an inflammation or quinsy [6, 7].

3.6.4 Surfaces

Medial surface is the free mucosal part of the tonsil that faces the oropharynx and contains bulging lymphoid projects. It is lined by stratified squamous nonkeratinized epithelium which contains polygonal superficial cells with microridges and numerous tubule-like long invaginations or orifices leading into tonsillar crypts. There are about 10–30 branching (primary and secondary) and anastomosing crypts, small pores, ranging in size between 5 and 25 μm. They increase the surface area of the tonsil up to 300 cm^2 except the anterior part for interactions between antigens and the nodular lymphoid tissue. Secondary crypts are branching part of the primary crypts and continue deeply into the lymphoid tissue and forms the lymphoid fronds. The largest and deepest crypt is called crypta magna or intratonsillar cleft which is localized near the upper part of the tonsil [6, 7, 9].

The transitional type nonkeratinized stratified epithelium, reticulated lymphoepithelium, with a discontinuous basement membrane covers the crypts with fenestrated capillaries and represents pores that are filled with large oval microvillus cells (M cells or dendritic cells) or lymphocytes (T and B cells). Dendritic cells play a role in the uptake and transport of antigens to extrafollicular T cell and B cell follicles [9, 12].

At about 5th month of gestation, there are no germinal centers, and the lymphocytes develop from the connective tissue cells or are relocated in the blood and lymph vessels [13]. After birth, the exogenous antigens cause immune response which is represented by the transformation of effector B cell into extrafollicular plasma cell in 2 weeks, and secondary follicles containing active germinal centers develop and rapidly expand not invade the surrounding tissue in the first decade of life [7, 12]. The tonsillar lymphoid follicles consist of the lymphoid (germinal centers) and non-lymphoid cells (reticular cells and dendritic cells/macrophages). The germinal center is composed of a central area of proliferating B cells which is surrounded by resting B and T cells. Between these follicles, high endothelial venules allow the entrance of T and B cells from the blood and the release of mature lymphocytes into blood [6, 9, 13]. So, the tonsils have efferent lymphatic vessels to connect to lymph nodes, but no afferent vessels unlike a lymph node. The lymphoid fronds are separated from the tonsillar bed by a capsule, which is firmly coherent to the lymphoid tissue by multiple septa or trabeculae that dissect the tonsillar parenchyma. The trabeculae consist of elastin fibers and reticular fibers that are composed of type III collagen and provide cytoskeletal support. So, each tonsil is in a fixed position, in contrast to other MALTs, which are distributed throughout the body, and to disconnect the tonsil from its capsule is impossible. Also, the nerves, lymphatic and blood vessels, pass through the trabeculae [6, 9, 12].

The tonsils are most immunologically active at 4–10 years of age, whereas the adenoids are at 4–6 years. Age-dependent involution of the tonsil which refers to the regression of the germinal centers and the proliferation of fibrous tissue including the capsule and trabeculae occurs by adolescence. Also, fat deposition in tonsils starts and increases after 25 years of age [12, 13].

Lateral surface is a base of the tonsil that is covered by well-defined fibrous capsule at the lateral wall of the tonsillar fossa, which is composed of five layers from within outward (**Figure 3**):

1. Tonsillar capsule, a thin false or surgical sheet, covers the tonsillar fossa as an appendage of the pharyngobasilar fascia. The upper part of this condensed

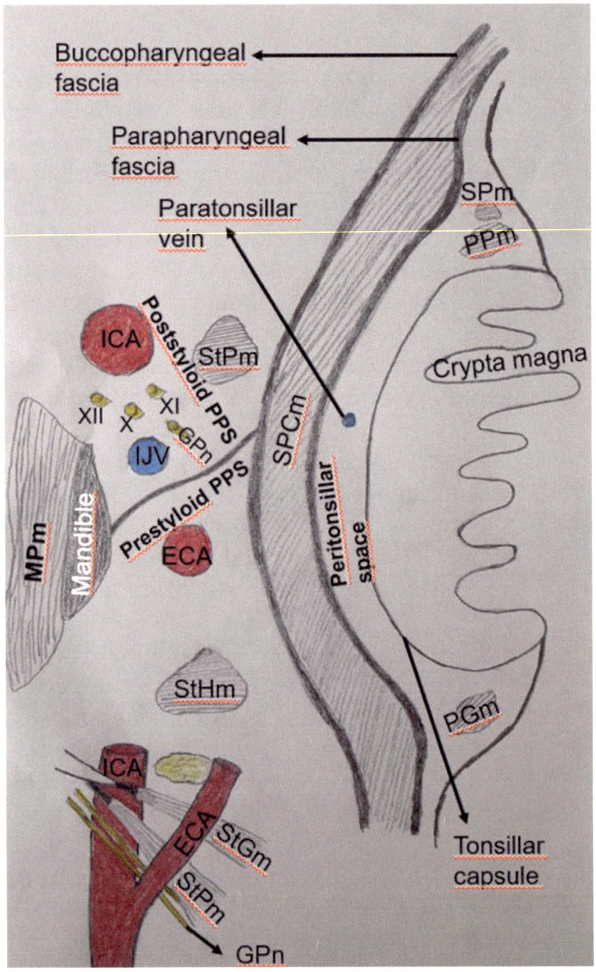

Figure 3.
The layers of the lateral pharyngeal wall at the level of tonsillar fossa, the parapharyngeal space compartments, and the structures between external and internal carotid arteries: SPm, salpingopharyngeus muscle; SPCm, superior pharyngeal constrictor muscle; PPm, palatopharyngeus muscle; PGm, palatoglossal muscle; StPm, stylopharyngeus muscle; StHm, stylohyoid muscle; StGm, styloglossus muscle; MPm, medial pterygoid muscle; GPn, glossopharyngeal nerve; PPS, parapharyngeal space; ICA, internal carotid artery; ECA, external carotid artery; X, vagus nerve; XI, accessory nerve; XII, hypoglossal nerve.

capsule is even and loosely fixed, whereas the lower part is irregular and intermingled with the pharyngeal muscle fibers and is firmly attached anteroinferiorly by the suspensory ligament to the posterior one third of the tongue. The tonsillar artery enters near this ligament. So, the surgical removal of the upper part of the capsule up to the lower third is very easy, but the lower part requires cautious resection [6, 7, 14].

2. Loose areolar tissue refers to the peritonsillar space between the tonsillar capsule and the pharyngobasilar fascia and contains the paratonsillar veins. A collection of pus in this space result in peritonsillar abscess or quinsy. It allows free movement of the pharyngeal muscles in the bed and makes easy to dissect the tonsil with capsule during tonsillectomy [6, 7].

3. Pharyngobasilar fascia or pharyngeal aponeurosis originates from the pharyngeal tubercle and covers the first layer of the SPCm and is limited with the

inferior fibers of the muscle. Efferent lymphatic vessels from the tonsil pierce through the buccopharyngeal fascia [7, 15].

4. The lateral wall of tonsillar fossa or tonsillar bed is mostly made up of the SPCm and pharyngobasilar fascia superiorly, the StPm posteriorly, and the stylohyoid ligament, middle pharyngeal constrictor (MPCm), the glossopharyngeal nerve (GPn), and styloglossus (StGm) muscles anteroinferiorly [7, 14, 15].

The SPCm narrows the superior part of the pharynx and is composed of four portions depending on their origins;

a. The pterygopharyngeal portion originates from the posterior margin of the medial pterygoid plate and pterygoid hamulus.

b. The buccopharyngeal portion arises from the pterygomandibular raphe.

c. The mylopharyngeal portion originates from the posterior end of the mylohyoid line of the mandible.

d. The glossopharyngeal portion arises from the side of the tongue.

All of the muscle fibers are inserted into the median pharyngeal raphe posteriorly [7, 11]. Frequently, there is a space of 1–3 cm between the SPCm and MPCm. The GPn between the stylohyoid ligament and StGm curve forward and medially and pass through this space at the level of the lower pole of the palatine tonsil. The StGm and stylohyoid ligament originate from the anterior margin of the styloid process near its apex. The StGm inserts into the inferolateral surface of the tongue and interdigitates with intrinsic longitudinal lingual muscle, whereas the stylohyoid ligament lies between the StPm and StGm and attaches to the hyoid bone medially [7, 11, 16]. The StGm functions to elevate and retract the base of the tongue. Inferolaterally the lingual artery crosses the StGm and gives the dorsal lingual branches medial to the attachment of the StGm to the base of tongue [16].

At the junction of pharyngeal constrictor muscles beneath the tonsil, the GPn gives tonsillar branch and afterward, extends into the base of tongue between the StGm and the stylohyoid ligament posteroinferiorly. The StPm originates from the posterior margin of the styloid process and courses downward along the posterolateral part of the stylohyoid ligament. Between the SPCm and MPCm, it passes and inserts to the PPm, MPCm, and pharyngeal mucosa [14, 17].

5. The buccopharyngeal fascia covers the lateral aspect of the SPCm medially and the medial pterygoid muscle anterolaterally. It forms anteromedial wall of the PPS and contains the pharyngeal plexus of nerves and vessels. The PPS like an inverted pyramid is situated between the lateral pharyngeal wall and the pterygoid musculature (**Figure 3**) [4, 15].

3.7 Anatomy of the parapharyngeal space

The base of the parapharyngeal pyramid is located at the skull base and its apex at the greater cornu of the hyoid bone. The PPS is bounded by the following structures:

a. The buccopharyngeal fascia which covers the SPCm, the LVPm, and tensor veli palatini muscles medially,

b. The fascia overlying the masticator space, the medial pterygoid muscle, the sphenomandibular ligament, the ramus of the mandible, and the deep lobe of the parotid gland anterolaterally,

c. The styloid process, the StGm and StPm posterolaterally,

d. The pterygomandibular raphe between the medial pterygoid plate and the mylohyoid line of the mandible and interpterygoid fascia anteriorly,

e. The prevertebral fascia and muscles posteriorly.

Inferiorly, the direct communication of the PPS with the submandibular space may be seen at the apex [4, 7, 10, 15].

3.7.1 Parapharyngeal space compartments

Prasad et al. reported that the PPS is composed of three compartments as follows: the upper part of the PPS is located between the skull base and the axial plane passing through the inferior border of the lateral pterygoid muscle, the lower border of the middle part is formed by the axial plane passing through the mandibular insertion of medial pterygoid muscle, and the lower part is limited with the hyoid bone. The middle part of the PPS is situated at the level of the tonsillar fossa. Also, the upper and middle parts are divided into prestyloid and poststyloid compartments in relation to the styloid diaphragm. Thus, the PPS consists of five parapharyngeal subspaces [18].

The styloid diaphragm is a thick gray fascia which is composed of the posterior belly of the digastric muscle, the styloid musculature (StPm, StGm and stylohyoid muscle-StHm), and the stylohyoid and stylomandibular ligaments. It divides the lower PPS into the prestyloid and poststyloid compartments by extending from the styloid process to the parotid fascia (**Figure 3**). The prestyloid space is localized between the medial pterygoid muscle and SPCm [7, 15, 18].

In the prestyloid part of the upper PPS, minor salivary glands, the posterior division of the mandibular nerve, the internal maxillary artery, fat pad, and tensor veli palatini muscle are located. In the poststyloid part of the upper PPS, the carotid sheath which consists of the internal carotid artery (ICA), internal jugular vein (IJV), vagus nerve, and also just in this superior section the ascending pharyngeal artery, cervical sympathetic chain, and the lower cranial nerves, IX, XI, and XII, are situated [7, 18].

In the prestyloid part of the middle PPS, the fat pad, a deep lobe of the parotid gland, from superior to inferior numerous tonsillar branches of the descending palatine, the ascending pharyngeal, and the ascending palatine arteries between the StGm and StPm are located. In the poststyloid part of the middle PPS, the curves of the internal maxillary, facial, and lingual arteries, cervical sympathetic chain, and the carotid sheath which consists of the ICA, IJV, and the lower cranial nerves (CNIX–CNXII) are situated [5, 7, 18].

3.7.2 Surgical landmarks in the parapharyngeal space in relation to the palatine tonsil

Different surgical procedures can be used in treatment of the upper airway obstruction due to tonsillar or adeno-tonsillar hypertrophy and peritonsillar abscess. Classic tonsillectomy consists of full removal of the tonsil with its capsule by dissecting the peritonsillar space with or without adenoidectomy. In the post-acute tonsillitis, a peritonsillar abscess may spread into the PPS through the buccopharyngeal fascia. Due to the close proximity of the PPS with the surrounding spaces including pharyngeal mucosal, retropharyngeal, masticator, and parotid spaces, the lesions in these spaces commonly spread into the PPS and result in secondary lesions [4, 5].

Sun et al. reported that the localization of the tumors in the PPS can be identified by some anatomical landmarks during surgical approaches. Because of the tumors in the upper PPS are mostly benign and located in the prestyloid space, the endoscopic transnasal transpterygoid approaches to this region require detailed anatomic knowledge of the surgical anatomic landmarks in this space. They demonstrated that the surgical anatomic landmarks in the prestyloid part of the upper PPS are as follows: the pterygoid process with medial and lateral plates, the tensor veli palatini, the SPCm, the lateral and medial pterygoid muscles, and the fat pad. In the prestyloid part of the lower PPS, the PGa, the SPCm, the pterygomandibular raphe, fat tissue, and the styloid diaphragm could be used as surgical anatomical landmarks during endoscopic transoral approach (**Figure 3**) [19].

Approximately 80% of primary oropharyngeal tumors originate from the tonsillar fossa and their incidence in younger patients increases. The tumors in the tonsillar fossa and the PPS can be removed by endoscope-assisted lateral oropharyngectomy approaches, transoral robotic surgery, or laser microsurgery. The lateral pharyngeal wall is composed of three deep fascia layers from inward to outward: the capsule of the tonsil, the pharyngobasilar fascia, and the buccopharyngeal fascia [5, 15, 19]. Depending on these fascia layers, De Virgilio et al. reported their lateral oropharyngectomy classification based on three types of surgical procedures and four possible extensions (superior, soft palate; posterior, pharyngeal wall; inferior, base of the tongue; anterior, retromolar trigone) [5].

Type 1 contains the removal of the palatine tonsil deep to the pharyngobasilar fascia with the resection of all or part of the anterior pillar excluding the SPCm. The aim of this procedure is mostly diagnostic, but it can be used in surgical treatment of noninvasive hyperplasia, dysplasia, or carcinoma in situ of the tonsil.

Type 2 is resection of the palatine tonsil, the PGm, the PPm, and the SPCm deep to the buccopharyngeal fascia. It can be therapeutic for invasive malignant tumors not grossly infiltrating the SPCm.

Type 3 includes the resection of the buccopharyngeal fascia with extension to the pterygoid muscle and PPS adipose corpus in addition to Type 2 contents. According to the extension of the tumor, the resection of the PPS tissue up to the exposure of the ICA could be included, and also a flap coverage for the ICA is required [5].

Similarly, Mirapeix et al. identified an applicable dissection method based on the anatomic stratification and evident anatomic landmarks [4]. They performed the dissections layer by layer from within outward and described this technique by dividing the lateral oropharyngeal wall into three layers:

The first layer, medial to styloid muscles, includes important surgical landmarks such as the SPCm, PGm, PPm, and StGm, the pharyngobasilar fascia, and a vascular network, which is composed of the branches of the descending and ascending palatine arteries and the ascending pharyngeal artery. The vascular supply of the tonsillar fossa can be identified by the PGm and PPm, and also the lingual branch of the GPn mostly crosses at the midpoint between PGm and PPm or along the posteroinferior edge of the StGm.

The second layer is observed after resection of the constrictor muscles and located in the PPS medial to the styloid diaphragm. The surgical landmarks are composed of the styloid musculature, the buccopharyngeal fascia, the stylohyoid ligament, the pharyngeal venous plexus, and the GPn. The insertion point of the

StGm refers to junction of the tongue with anterior pillar, and the lingual branch of the GPn can be identified along the posteroinferior border of the StGm. The pharyngeal venous plexus is located in a space between the StGm and SPCm. The facial artery and the hypoglossal nerve cross the StHm which extends parallel to the stylohyoid ligament. The GPn travels downward along the posterolateral aspect of the StPm.

The third layer lateral to styloid diaphragm refers to the poststyloid part of the PPS. Surgical landmarks in this layer consist of the styloid musculature, the posterior belly of the digastric muscle, the ICA, the hypoglossal nerve, and lingual and facial arteries. Especially, the StGm is an essential landmark to identify the localization of the ICA posterolaterally, the lingual nerve anteriorly, and the submandibular gland inferolaterally. The hypoglossal nerve crosses laterally to medially over the ascending pharyngeal originating from the superolateral border of the external carotid artery (ECA) in the poststyloid part of the lower PPS [4].

During transoral robotic surgery (TORS), the dissection of the SPCm from the pterygomandibular raphe refers to a window into the prestyloid compartment of the PPS. The tendon of the medial pterygoid muscle leads to identification of the buccopharyngeal fascia and indicates a safe plane in the prestyloid compartment of the PPS [7, 19]. Also, the plane that is constituted by the styloid musculature and the stylohyoid ligament is an essential surgical landmark for ICA identification. Wang et al. demonstrated that the styloid process, styloid diaphragm, pharyngeal venous plexus, GPn, and pharyngeal branch of the vagus are located between the ECA and the ICA and subdivide the PPS into prestyloid and poststyloid spaces (**Figure 3**). The curves of the branches of the ECA (lingual, facial, ascending pharyngeal, internal maxillary arteries) are located in the prestyloid space, and also the ascending pharyngeal artery crosses the StGm at the distal third near the tonsillar fossa surgical field [20]. In addition, the lingual artery and hypoglossal nerve are located lateral to the StGm, and the lingual artery passes between greater cornu of hyoid and the StGm where it has high risk of hemorrhage during the resection of the base of the tongue [21]. The fact that in the PPS the facial artery is located inferolateral to the StGm is of great importance, because a dissection lateral to the StGm or resection of tonsillar malignancy may result in significant hemorrhage. In PPS after branching from the facial artery, the tonsillar and ascending palatine arteries course between the StGm and the StPm and then pierce the SPCm to supply the tonsil [22]. So, the fact that the StGm is in close relationship with the branches of the ECA should be kept in mind when the transoral dissection space at the level of the tonsillar fossa is dissected in the superolateral direction, and the dissection deep into the plane of this muscle must be performed rigorously and accurately [16, 20].

In the PPS lateral to the styloid diaphragm, the ICA lies about 10–20 mm behind the palatine tonsil at the level of the epiglottis apex, whereas its distance to the ET is approximately 23.5 mm. So, it is closer to the lateral pharyngeal wall in the poststyloid part of the lower PPS than in the upper PPS, and the risk of arterial trauma during tonsillectomy increases with a decrease in the distance to the pharyngeal wall. Also, the level of the common carotid artery bifurcation higher than the epiglottis apex is more susceptible to common carotid artery trauma during surgery [23]. During radical tonsillectomy, because the lingual nerve lies lateral to the SPCm, it may be injured at the anterior border of the medial pterygoid muscle [15].

The GPn extends from the jugular foramen to the base of the tongue in the lateral wall of the pharynx. Because of the close relationship of the GPn with the StPm, it is divided into three parts: upper (jugular foramen, upper border of the StPm), middle (upper-lower borders of the StPm), and lower (lower borders of the StPm, the base of the tongue) [17].

The upper part travels between the ICA and IJV behind the styloid process and gives the carotid body and carotid sinus branches in the poststyloid part of the upper PPS.

The middle part extends downward along the inferolateral border of the StPm and gives off branches to the StPm and pharyngeal wall in the poststyloid part of the lower PPS. Particularly, this part passes obliquely anterior to the distal segment of the ICA and may result in vascular injury.

The lower part passes through a space or slit between the SPCm and MPCm to enter the pharynx. Between the StGm and StPm, it lies along the inferior border of the palatine tonsil or beneath the capsule and gives the tonsillar branch. Generally, it gives terminal branches at the junction of the PPa with the base of tongue, known as glossotonsillar sulcus, which is anatomic landmark for the terminal part of the GPn deep to the SPCm [17].

During surgical interventions including transoral tonsillectomy, tumor resection, and the SPCm block, the integrity of this nerve may be damaged and result in dysphagia and taste disturbance. In recurrent tonsillitis, the adherence of the capsule with surrounding structures makes it difficult to remove the hypertrophic tonsillar capsule from the tonsillar bed, or the dissection of the capsule which is firmly adherent with the lingual branch of this nerve causes disturbance of the nerve functions [3, 7, 17]. During transoral surgery, early description of the StPm allows to specify the GPn which crosses over the ICA and serves as a surgical landmark to protect it in the PPS. Also, the surgeon should keep in mind the association of the GPn with a venous plexus in the glossotonsillar sulcus to prevent iatrogenic bleeding during surgical dissection.

3.8 Vascular network and innervation of the tonsils

3.8.1 Arterial supply

The tonsil and tonsillar fossa with boundaries are supplied by the branches of the ECA including lingual, facial, ascending pharyngeal, and internal maxillary arteries (**Figure 4**).

The upper part is supplied by descending palatine artery branch of the internal maxillary artery and the middle and inferior branches of the ascending pharyngeal artery.

The middle part is supplied by tonsillar branch of the facial artery.

The lower part is supplied by an ascending palatine artery branch of the facial artery and dorsal lingual branch of the lingual artery [20, 23].

3.8.2 Venous drainage

The veins of the tonsil and tonsillar fossa drain into the paratonsillar vein and then into the pharyngeal venous plexus. This plexus drains through the facial vein into the IJV (**Figure 4**) [6, 7].

3.8.3 Lymphatic drainage

The lymphatics pierce the SPCm and drain into the upper deep cervical lymph nodes principally jugulodigastric lymph nodes which are located below the angle of the mandible posteriorly [6, 7].

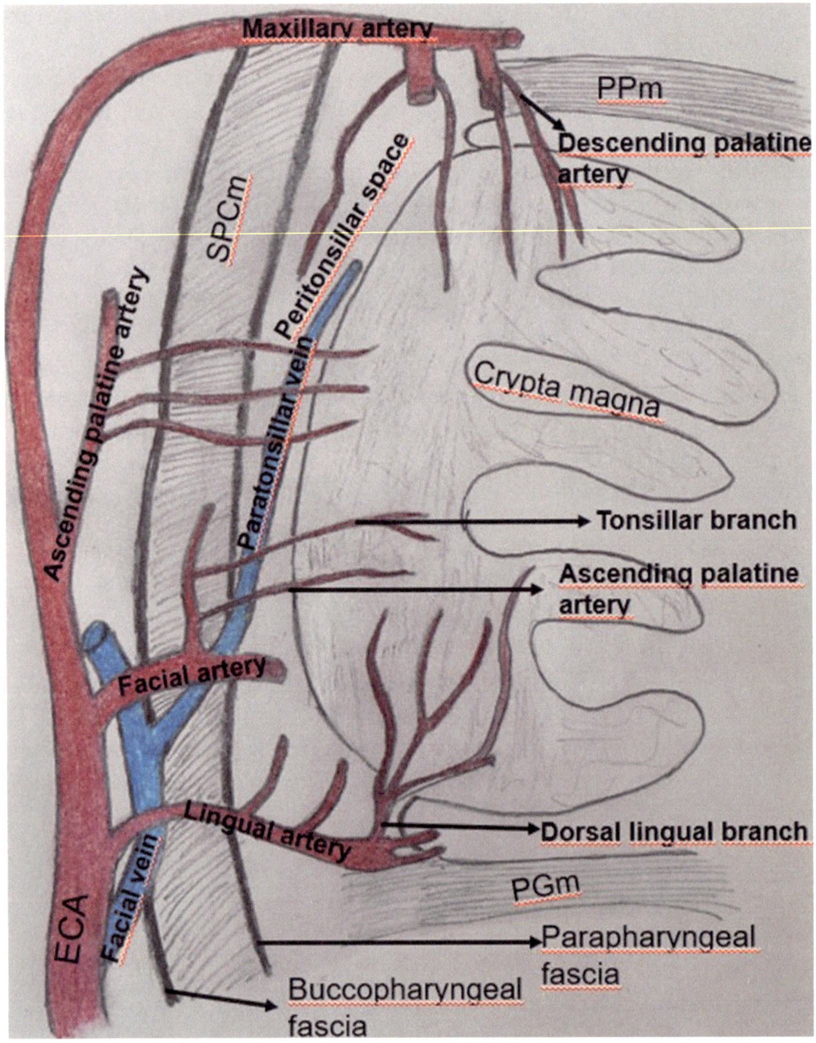

Figure 4.
The vascular supply of the tonsil: PPm, palatopharyngeus muscle; PGm, palatoglossal muscle; SPCm, superior pharyngeal constrictor muscle.

3.8.4 Nerve supply

General sensation of the tonsil and tonsillar fossa is supplied by the tonsillar branches of the GPn and the lesser palatine branch of the pterygopalatine ganglion (the maxillary division of the trigeminal nerve) [6, 7].

4. Conclusions

Benign or malign lesions in the tonsil and tonsillar fossa may penetrate the lateral wall of the pharynx, or the PPS may be distorted evidently by the tumors. Due to the anatomical complexity with vital neurovascular structures in the PPS, transoral robotic approach to this region makes it necessary to identify the surgical anatomic landmarks which are required to perform effective surgical intervention quickly and accurately. The detailed and precise anatomic knowledge of the tonsillar region and the PPS allows surgeon to carry out wide resections in a confined space. In transoral approaches, the classification of the dissection method based on the anatomic stratification or the surgical procedures which is oriented to cardinal points is essential for preoperative planning and to prevent the iatrogenic complications.

Conflict of interest

The author reports no conflict of interest concerning the materials used in this paper. And the author has no personal financial or institutional interest in this article.

Author details

Gülay Açar
Necmettin Erbakan University, Meram Faculty of Medicine, Department of Anatomy, Konya, Turkey

*Address all correspondence to: gulayzeynep73@gmail.com

References

[1] Ruddle NH, Akirav EM. Secondary lymphoid organs: Responding to genetic and environmental cues in ontogeny and the immune response. Journal of Immunology. 2009;**183**(4):2205-2212. DOI: 10.4049/jimmunol.0804324 Review

[2] Masieri S, Trabattoni D, Incorvaia C, De Luca MC, Dell'Albani I, Leo G, et al. A role for Waldeyer's ring in immunological response to allergens. Current Medical Research and Opinion. 2014;**30**(2):203-205. DOI: 10.1185/03007995.2013.855185

[3] Masters KG, Lasrado S. Anatomy, Head and Neck, Tonsils. StatPearls [Internet]. Treasure Island (FL): StatPearls Publishing; 2020

[4] Mirapeix RM, Tobed Secall M, Pollán Guisasola C, Garcia Lorenzo J, Lluansí Planella J, Viña Soria C, et al. Anatomic landmarks in transoral oropharyngeal surgery. The Journal of Craniofacial Surgery. 2019;**30**(2):e101-e106. DOI: 10.1097/SCS.0000000000004935

[5] De Virgilio A, Kim SH, Magnuson JS, Holsinger C, Remacle M, Lawson G, et al. Anatomical-based classification for transoral lateral oropharyngectomy. Oral Oncology. 2019;**99**:104450. DOI: 10.1016/j.oraloncology.2019.104450

[6] Regauer S. Nasopharynx and Waldeyer's ring. In: Cardesa A, Slootweg PJ, editors. Pathology of the Head & Neck. New York: Springer; 2006. pp. 183-189.ch6

[7] Brodsky L, Poje C. Tonsillitis, tonsillectomy, and adenoidectomy. In: Bailey BJ, Johnson JT, Newlands SD, editors. Head and Neck Surgery -Otolaryngology. 4th ed. Philadelphia: Lippincott Williams & Wilkins; 2006. pp. 1183-1195

[8] Fukino K, Tsutsumi M, Sanudo J, Ono T, Akita K. Anatomical significance of the spatial distribution of the palatopharyngeus with regard to velopharyngeal closure. The Cleft Palate-Craniofacial Journal. 2019;**56**(6):744-750. DOI: 10.1177/1055665618813082

[9] Fossum CC, Chintakuntlawar AV, Price DL, Garcia JJ. Characterization of the oropharynx: Anatomy, histology, immunology, squamous cell carcinoma and surgical resection. Histopathology. 2017;**70**(7):1021-1029. DOI: 10.1111/his.13140

[10] Goyal N, Yoo F, Goldenberg D. Oropharyngeal anatomy and radical tonsillectomy. In: Goldenberg D, Goyal N, editors. Robotic Head and Neck Surgery: An Anatomical and Surgical Atlas. 1st ed. New York, Stuttgart: Thieme Publishers; 2017. pp. 1-4. DOI: 10.1055/b-0038-149746.ch1

[11] Sakamoto Y. Spatial relationship between the palatopharyngeus and the superior constrictor of the pharynx. Surgical and Radiologic Anatomy. 2015;**37**(6):649-655. DOI: 10.1007/s00276-015-1444-5

[12] Isaacson G, Parikh T. Developmental anatomy of the tonsil and its implications for intracapsular tonsillectomy. International Journal of Pediatric Otorhinolaryngology. 2008;**72**(1):89-96

[13] Noussios G, Xanthopoulos J, Zaraboukas T, Vital V, Konstantinidis I. Morphological study of development and functional activity of palatine tonsils in embryonic age. Acta Otorhinolaryngologica. 2003;**23**(2):98-101

[14] Ohtsuka K, Tomita H, Murakami G. Anatomy of the tonsillar bed: Topographical relationship between the palatine tonsil and the lingual branch of

the glossopharyngeal nerve. Acta Oto-Laryngologica. 2002;**546**:99-109

[15] Gun R, Durmus K, Kucur C, Carrau RL, Ozer E. Transoral surgical anatomy and clinical considerations of lateral oropharyngeal wall, parapharyngeal space, and tongue base. Otolaryngology and Head and Neck Surgery. 2016;**154**(3):480-485. DOI: 10.1177/0194599815625911

[16] Laccourreye O, Orosco RK, Rubin F, Holsinger FC. Styloglossus muscle: A critical landmark in head and neck oncology. European Annals of Otorhinolaryngology, Head and Neck Diseases. 2018;**135**(6):421-425. DOI: 10.1016/j.anorl.2017.11.012 Review

[17] Wang C, Kundaria S, Fernandez-Miranda J, Duvvuri U. A description of the anatomy of the glossopharyngeal nerve as encountered in transoral surgery. Laryngoscope. 2016;**126**(9):2010-2015. DOI: 10.1002/lary.25706

[18] Prasad SC, Piccirillo E, Chovanec M, La Melia C, De Donato G, Sanna M. Lateral skull base approaches in the management of benign parapharyngeal space tumors. Auris Nasus Larynx. 2015;**42**(3):189-198

[19] Sun X, Yan B, Truong HQ, Borghei-Razavi H, Snyderman CH, Fernandez-Miranda JC. A comparative analysis of endoscopic-assisted transoral and transnasal approaches to parapharyngeal space: A cadaveric study. Journal of Neurological Surgery B Skull Base. 2018;**79**(3):229-240. DOI: 10.1055/s-0037-1606551

[20] Wang C, Kundaria S, Fernandez-Miranda J, Duvvuri U. A description of arterial variants in the transoral approach to the parapharyngeal space. Clinical Anatomy. 2014;**27**(7):1016-1022. DOI: 10.1002/ca.22273

[21] Gun R, Ozer E. Surgical anatomy of oropharynx and supraglottic larynx for transoral robotic surgery. Journal of Surgical Oncology. 2015;**112**(7):690-696. DOI: 10.1002/jso.24020 Review

[22] Mohamed A, Paleri V, George A. A cadaveric study quantifying the anatomical landmarks of the facial artery and its parapharyngeal branches for safe transoral surgery. Head & Neck. 2019;**41**(9):3389-3394. DOI: 10.1002/hed.25862

[23] Zając HJ, Lachowski K, Lis A, Kręcicki T, Garcarek J, Guziński M, et al. The anatomical relation of the extracranial internal carotid artery in the parapharyngeal space. Advances in Clinical and Experimental Medicine. 2019;**28**(5):601-607. DOI: 10.17219/acem/78350

Chapter 3

Methods of Collection and Transport of Materials to Laboratory from Oral and Dental Tissue Lesions

Krishna Sireesha Sundaragiri, Soumya Makarla and Bharat Sankhla

Abstract

The oral pathology laboratory is the most resourceful place for the diagnosis of oral lesions. Most clinicians err on the collection and transport of oral and associated tissues to the laboratory. Oral tissue examination includes a wide range such as oral biopsy (for routine formalin fixed and fresh tissue), saliva, swabs, cytology smears and fine needle-aspirated, cystic fluid. This in turn adversely affects the final diagnosis of the disease. Thus, it is high time to appreciate and acknowledge the role of collection containers, fixing reagents and transport media as an adjunct for successful diagnosis.

Keywords: oral, biopsy, saliva, cytology, laboratory

1. Introduction

The role of the general as well as oral pathology and microbiology laboratory is essential to the successful provision of patient care. Appropriate, professional and knowledgeable interaction with the dental or head and neck surgeon can benefit the patients by achieving accurate diagnosis as well as effective treatment approaches. Acquiring proper laboratory data allows the dental practitioner to arrive at a definitive diagnosis for further referral in a timely manner as oral cavity often presents the first signs of a systemic illness. The pathologist plays a valuable role in education and documentation of the learned information for future cases with similar presentation for he/she presents the final verdict.

The oral pathology laboratory is the most resourceful place for the diagnosis of oral lesions. A multitude of lesions are encountered in the oral and maxillofacial regions that need a sound knowledge of how to approach their diagnosis, and it begins with a good clinical history and examination. The basic requirements of a useful diagnostic technique are ease of use, patient acceptance and sufficient specimen collection. The ideal diagnostic procedure should also be highly sensitive and specific, simple, and not time-consuming and have a potential for automation [1]. Oral tissue examination includes a wide range such as oral biopsy (for routine formalin fixed and fresh tissue), saliva, swabs, cytology smears and fine needle-aspirated, cystic fluid and microbiology.

IntechOpen

2. Biopsy: rationale

When a patient with a particular lesion is seen, a list of differential diagnosis is formulated, and biopsy is useful at arriving at a definitive diagnosis or to confirm the clinical diagnosis. Oral biopsy was and still is the gold standard for oral diagnostic procedures. It is an invasive procedure with procedural limitations and a psychological effect on patients. It is important that the biopsy specimen be a true representation of the entire lesion. A carefully selected area involving normal as well as pathologic areas can produce good diagnostic specimen.

2.1 Dos and Don'ts for sample collection

1. Take tissue specimen, and put it into a wide-mouth container with 10% formalin at least 20 times the volume of the surgical specimen. Care should be taken to be sure that the tissue has not become lodged on the wall of the container above the level of the formalin.

2. Incisional biopsy specimens should be taken from each area showing different characteristics. Even if the lesion clinically looks uniform, it is still wise to sample different areas of a large lesion. Multiple samples must be adequately labeled.

3. Vigorous manipulation of lesion should be avoided if it is suspected to be tumor as it can increase the tumor cell emboli in venous drainage.

4. The tissue should never be put on gauze, cotton or paper, as it can lead to dehydration of the tissue specimen.

5. If culture is desired, take the material for bacteriologic study before fixing the specimen.

6. On the other hand, if the lesion is a large one with variations in its clinical appearance multiple biopsies could be planned for better sampling.

7. Even though the pathologist would like to receive the biggest specimen possible, the minimum size of the biopsy should not be less than 5 mm in diameter, to enable the pathologist to obtain well-prepared slides.

8. In majority of cases, the most active part of the lesion and, therefore, the most representative are located peripherally. If the biopsy specimen is taken from a necrotic part of the tumor, the diagnosis rendered by the oral pathologist can be only the "necrotic tissue." Therefore, as a rule, it is unwise to biopsy the center of a lesion, which is probably its least active part [2, 3].

3. Tissue fixation

It is extremely important to place the biopsy specimen into proper fixative immediately after removal from the patient. Ten percent formalin is the standard fixative used to prevent autolysis, distortion and destruction of the tissues. Most oral pathology laboratories will provide mailing containers, specimen bottles filled with 10% formalin, and history-biopsy request sheet. **Table 1** is a list of fixatives with reference to oral tissue.

	Name	Composition	Comments
For routine histopathology	Phosphate buffered formalin	40% formaldehyde with Sodium dihydrogen phosphate monohydrate & disodium hydrogen phosphate anhydrous. pH - 6.8 Fixation time: 12 – 24 hours	Antigen retrival of successful IHC
	Formal calcium	40% formaldehyde & Calcium chloride Fixation time: 12 – 24 hours	for the preservation of lipids especially phospholipids.
	Formal saline	40% formaldehyde & Sodium chloride Fixation time: 12 – 24 hours	Widely used for routine histopathology prior to the introduction of phosphate buffered formalin. Often produces formalin pigment.
	Zinc formalin (unbuffered)	Zinc sulphate: 1 g 40% formaldehyde Fixation time: 4 – 8 hours	Alternatives to mercuric chloride formulations. Improved results with IHC
	Zenker's fixative	Mercuric chloride: 50 g Potassium dichromate: 25 g Glacial acetic acid: 50 ml in 950mL distilled water. Fixation time: 4 – 24 hours	Good nuclear preservation but lyses red blood cells (recommended for congested specimens) Gives good results with PTAH and trichrome staining. Produces mercury pigment
			which should be removed from sections prior to staining and can produce chrome pigment if tissue is not washed in water prior to processing. Is an intolerant agent so, after water washing, tissue should be stored in 70% ethanol.
	Helly's fixative	Potassium dichromate: 25 g Sodium sulphate: 10 g Mercuric chloride: 50 g Immediately before use add – 40% formaldehyde Fixation time: 4 – 24 hours	
	B-5 fixative	B-5 fixative prepare immediately before use Sodium sulphate: 10 g Mercuric chloride: 50 g Immediately before use add – 40% formaldehyde: 50 ml Fixation time: 4 – 24 hours	Fixation of haematopoietic and lymphoid tissue. It produces excellent nuclear detail, provides good results with many special stains and is recommended for IHC.
	Carnoy's solution	Ethanol absolute: 60 ml Chloroform: 30 ml Acetic acid glacial: 10 ml Fixation time: 1 – 4 hours	Is rapid acting, gives good nuclear preservation and retains glycogen

Table 1.
List of fixatives with reference to oral tissue.

3.1 Precautions

a. If the fixative in the mailing container has evaporated, leaving a white powder residue, it cannot be reconstituted by adding water.

b. Another container must be used or the fixative prepared by getting formalin (formaldehyde 37–40%) and mixing 10 parts of formalin solution with 100 parts of tap water.

c. The biopsy specimen must not dry out on the bracket table while one is finding the fixative, bottles and the like.

d. Everything should be ready in advance so that the tissues can be properly fixed and a diagnosis can be rendered and to avoid the statement "improper fixation, unable to render diagnosis."

e. The biopsy specimen should never be submitted in normal saline or water, as the tissues become completely degenerated by autolysis.

f. In an emergency, when 10% formalin cannot be obtained, 70% alcohol may be used. Alcohol causes hardening of the specimen to the degree that cutting may be difficult, so on the biopsy request form it should be noted that the specimen is submitted in alcohol. The histology technician can then transfer the specimen to 10% formalin, hopefully before 48 h, so that the tissue will not become too hard to cut.

g. Preserving the specimen. The specimen—a tooth, piece of bone, or soft tissue—is at once placed in a bottle containing a fixing solution, such as 10% formalin, Zenker's solution, or Carnoy's solution. Most pathologists prefer 10% formalin solution.

h. It should be promptly sent to a pathologist for examination. The latter should be given all the information gained by clinical study and X-ray examination, or other laboratory tests, as this will facilitate diagnosis in difficult cases.

i. A consultation between the pathologist and the dentist will be particularly helpful and will also give the opportunity for discussing the method of procedure in the treatment of the patient.

j. It is also very important that the completed history form be sent with the biopsy specimen [3].

3.1.1 Precautions during transport: freezing

During winter months in climates where the temperature drops to freezing or below, there is a danger that the biopsy specimens dropped in a mailbox may freeze. The freezing of the tissue forms ice crystals within the cells. These crystals disrupt cell membranes and cause great distortion and introduction of artifacts into the specimen. Thus interpretation of the tissue specimen becomes very tenuous.

Before mailing biopsy specimens during cold weather, one must make sure that they are fixed in 10% formalin at room temperature for at least 2 h before mailing.

3.1.2 Adjunct techniques: electrocautery

Biopsy specimens can display tissue changes that might interfere with the accurate diagnosis by the use of electrocautery. The frying action of the electric current generating high temperatures in the tissues results in changes.

In the case of a biopsy of an oral mucosa lesion, an eosinophilic homogenization of the fibrous tissue can be seen histologically. Thus, it is especially important not to use electrocautery for excision of small lesions. It is preferable to use a surgical scalpel to remove the biopsy specimen followed by the use of electrocautery to control bleeding [3].

3.2 Oral exfoliative cytology

Oral exfoliative cytology was developed as a potential diagnostic tool for early detection of malignant lesion. It is relatively simple, easy to master and least invasive and has high patient acceptance [1]. Though it has been always used as an adjunct to oral biopsy in oral cancer diagnostics, it holds potential in diagnosis of oral dermatosis and certain microbial infections. The specimen obtained can be used for cytomorphometry, DNA cytometry and immunocytochemical studies [1].

3.3 Technique: collection of smear

a. Toluidine blue should be used as a supravital stain before the site selection and smear preparation.

b. Label one end of the slide with patient's name, date, and area from which material is to be obtained. Wipe the slide clean.

c. Use a clean cotton tip applicator or wooden spatula for the collection of the smear. If the area to be scraped is dry, moistened the applicator or spatula.

d. Collect the material using a slight rolling motion or scraping of the lesion. (Inadequate slides may be obtained if there is a pseudomembrane, thick saliva, no moisture or excess bleeding).

e. Immediately apply the scraping to the center area of the slide previously marked.

3.3.1 Fixation of smear

a. Alcohol (70%) is adequate for fixation. Equal parts of ether and 95% ethyl alcohol give superior staining qualities.

b. Immediately immerse the slide in fixative or put the fixative on the slide with a dropper. Do not allow any drying of the smear before fixation.

c. Keep the slide in fixative for a minimum of 30 min.

d. At this point, the slides can be air dried and sent for staining and screening, or it can be left in the fixative.

Pt's name Site Date		C-

3.3.2 Advantages

a. Very good, easy, rapid, painless and bloodless procedure.

b. Adjunct to biopsy, better to take cytology first, and then if necessary advice biopsy.

c. Creates less psychological trauma and fear.

d. Useful in follow-up after radio- and chemotherapy.

e. Recurrence can be known very easily without taking biopsy.

f. Mainly used for ulcerative epithelial lesion; intact epithelium gives false negative result.

g. Also used for dermatological condition like pemphigus vulgaris, Darier's disease, and viral infections like herpes simplex as well as aphthous ulcers, etc.

Deeper lesions are not identified by this technique, and for that another technique called fine needle aspiration cytology (FNAC) is used.

4. Fine needle aspiration cytology

Fine needle aspiration biopsy or cytology is an effective tool in evaluating and diagnosing suspect lumps or masses. The name indicates this biopsy technique uses aspiration to obtain cells or fluid from a superficial or deep palpable mass. A quick diagnosis means that tumor is detected early, or benign lumps are diagnosed without the need for multiple surgeries [4]. The success of perfect FNAC depends on the technique for collection and preparation of samples along with a detailed clinical history and clinical impression. If an infectious process is suspected, often a portion of the specimen is submitted for microbiology in an appropriate sterile medium or transport container.

FNAC is indicated in head and neck lesions, which include salivary gland lesions, thyroid and parathyroid lesions, cervical lymph nodes and intraosseous lesions.

4.1 Collection: preparation for FNAC

Alcohol wipe; 4 × 4-inch gauze pads; 10-ml plastic syringes; 25-gauge 1 1/2-inch stiff, noncutting, bevel-edged needles; glass slides; alcohol bottles; pistol-grip mechanical syringe holder.

Procedure:

1. Explanation of procedure to the patient before doing FNAC ensures the patient's cooperation.

2. For head and neck biopsies, a chair with head rest is essential.

3. Prebiopsy sedation is usually not required, except in the deep aspirations in very anxious patients or for deep biopsies.

4. The patient is placed in a comfortable position—with mass readily palpable and easily graspable.

5. The lesion is grasped with one hand usually between two fingers with an attempt to determine the location and surrounding tissue.

6. The syringe pistol with attached needle is laid against the surface of the lesion at determined puncture site and angle.

7. The needle is inserted quickly and advanced into the mass.

8. The suction is applied to syringe, about one third the length of syringe barrel observing the junction of the hub and needle for appearance of any specimen.

9. Multiple short 5-mm "in-and-out" motions are made till tissue material is seen coming into the hub of the needle.

10. At first appearance of any sample at junction, the syringe pistol is released, letting the vacuum equate to normal, and the needle is withdrawn slowly.

11. Pressure is applied to the puncture site with sterile gauze pad.

12. The above procedure can be repeated again using a clean needle for a second pass (and more passes if needed).

4.2 Preparing the aspirate: making direct smears

The needle is removed quickly from the syringe. Five milliliters of air is aspirated into the syringe, and the needle is placed back on the syringe. With the needle bevel facing down, 1–2 drop of aspirated material is expelled onto each of several marked glass slides.

Preparation of smear: A drop of aspirate is placed at the center of plain glass slide. A second slide is inverted over the drop, and the slides are gently pulled apart vertically or horizontally once. Fix immediately in 95% ethyl alcohol for a wet smear. For studying and evaluating cytoplasmic features or background elements of smear, air drying is preferred. Until all the material in the needle is used, continue making more slides. Or a drop is placed near the frosted end of slide held in the left hand; the bloody material is spread along the edge of the slide held in the right hand. The material is pulled gently down the slide in a manner of making a blood smear.

Alternatively the expressed specimen is sent directly to the laboratory in a 50% ethyl alcohol fixative or Hank's balanced salt solution for slide preparation. If a cyst is aspirated, the laboratory will have to spin the specimen for concentration.

Modifications:

1. Often needle biopsy without aspiration based on capillary pressure in a fine needle is sufficient to keep the scraped cells inside the lumen. A 25-gauge needle is held directly with finger tips and is inserted into the target lesion and is moved back and forth in various directions. This procedure offers the advantage of better feel of tissue consistency and less admixture of blood and is valuable for tiny lymph nodes.

2. Cell block preparation: It refers to formalin fixing and paraffin embedding of aspiration biopsy that help reinforce some tissue patterns that may be seen on smears—aids in specific diagnosis especially for immunoperoxidase cytology staining.

3. Flow cytometry, electron microscopy and molecular diagnostic studies such as ELISA and FISH can be performed on FNAC specimens.

Storage instructions: Refrigerate in a fixative if there is delay.

Causes for rejection: Improper labeling, improper fixation and air-drying artifact.

5. Collection of specimen from cervical lymph nodes

The cervical and supraclavicular lymph nodes of the neck are in the drainage path of many infectious and malignant diseases; an examination should be made by

FNAC. FNAC of cervical lymph nodes is a well-accepted diagnostic test of choice in both adult and pediatric patients for reliably distinguishing between benign/reactive and malignant processes and guiding patient management with simple observation or antimicrobial therapy for infections, chemotherapy and radiation therapy or the need for more sample tissue like core biopsies or excisional biopsy of the lymph node itself [5].

Thus FNAC is recommended as a safe, quick and inexpensive tool in the diagnosis of head and neck lesions.

5.1 Saliva

Collection of human saliva offers a noninvasive method for monitoring the disposition of unbound (free) drugs and many endogenous biomarkers. Human genomic DNA extracted from buccal epithelial cells and white blood cells found in saliva can be used in various applications in diagnostics. The correlations between blood and saliva biomolecule/biomarker concentrations range from good to excellent. Methods of collecting saliva range from simply spitting into a collection cup or using absorbent pads or swabs or the trademarked collecting devices. Freeze-thaw techniques are often employed to help break up the mucin protein that is responsible for the sticky, foamy saliva. There are few inherent drawbacks for using saliva as an ideal biofluid. In some cases, the drug, metabolites or other compounds being assayed may bind to absorbent materials, thus reducing recovery or giving a misleading result [6].

Saliva is useful for testing:

a. As an index to metabolic processes

b. For caries activity tests

c. For detection of various metabolites in smokers

5.2 Collection of specimens

Whole saliva is commonly collected by draining, spitting, suction, and swab or absorbent method. Common stimuli used are chewing on paraffin wax and chewing gum at a fixed rate. As described by Wong D, the proposal for standardized collection of whole and glandular saliva can be followed for saliva sample collection.

1. Collect saliva samples at the same time of the day between 9:00 and 11:00 a.m.

2. Patient should refrain from eating and drinking at least 90 min before advised collection.

3. If present, drug usage should be stopped that might affect salivary secretion for at least 1 day.

4. Rinse mouth with preferably deionized water prior to the saliva collection.

5. Collect saliva for 10 min [6].

Collection of saliva into ice-cooled vials is recommended to slow down the activity of hydrolytic enzymes present in saliva in air-cooled preset environment. Proprietary collection vials contain a cocktail of protease inhibitors and bacteriostatic chemicals. Bacteria and cellular debris have to be removed directly after collection by centrifugating for 5 min at 10,000 g, or 20 min at 3000 g or by non-cotton-based filtration or vortexing (2 min, maximal speed).

6. Storage and transport

After collection, salivary samples must be snapped frozen in liquid nitrogen. In the absence of liquid nitrogen, freezing in dry ice is a practical choice when samples are collected. For a prolonged storage, −80°C temperature is preferred over storage at−20°C. The salivary samples can be diluted with glycerol (1:1) before storage. For immunochemical analysis such as ELISA, the saliva can be stored frozen after dilution (e.g., 1:100) in the assay buffer, usually PBS—0.5% Tween-20. To maintain the integrity of the proteins, before testing, the deep-frozen samples must be thawed as quickly as possible. Analysis of pH (H^+ and HCO_4^-) and viscoelastic properties is best analyzed in fresh saliva samples. Storage of salivary DNA and RNA is similar to that of a salivary protein sample [6].

7. Culture and sensitivity tests

Rationale: The idea of culturing microorganisms is not new or foreign to the practice of dentistry. There are situations in dentistry where it is not only important to know whether microorganisms are present in a lesion but also the type of microorganism. It follows from this that to best treat these infections the dentist needs to know what antibiotic would be most effective against the particular organism. Thus the culture and sensitivity test for bacterial organism is indispensable [7]. The biggest challenge today will be the transition from culture-based microbiological testing to molecular-based testing.

7.1 Collection of specimen

a. The success of oral bacteriologic/fungal identification procedures depends to a great extent on the manner in which the specimen is collected.

b. Lack of care and faulty methods of collection and handling of the specimen make the laboratory procedures valueless.

c. Because most of the microorganisms encountered in dental or head and neck infections are caused by facultative anaerobic or obligate anaerobic bacteria, the laboratory may prefer the use of a reducing transport media.

7.2 Tissue specimen for culture

a. The biopsy for culture is similar to the surgical biopsy for tissue diagnosis. A 5 × 5 × 5-mm piece of tissue is excised from the lesion with aseptic technique (here, it is undesirable to biopsy the normal tissue border, as there will not be any organisms in the normal tissues).

b. The biopsy specimen is placed in a sterile test tube containing sterile physiologic saline as the transport media (formalin is not used). The cap is secured and the specimen sent to the laboratory, along with the completed history sheet request form.

c. At the laboratory, using the sterile tissue grinders, the specimen is ground into suspension, which is left to settle. The supernatant fluid is then used for the inoculation of appropriate media [8].

8. Oral bacteriologic examination

8.1 Oral bacterial smears

For examination of surface lesions or exudates from a fistula or cyst, a specimen is procured by the means of a sterile platinum wire or a sterile exploring point. A sample of deposit or plaque on a tooth is gathered by the platinum loop, by exploring point or by a pipette. Root canal specimens may be taken with a sterile point. The specimen is then smeared on a glass slide. It is allowed to dry in the air and is fixed on the slide by drawing it three times through a Bunsen flame, when it is ready to be stained. For the proper collection of specimens, the precautions are:

a. Do not use antiseptic or disinfectants for cleaning the site from which the culture specimen is taken; just dry the site with sterile gauze.

b. The sterile swab moistened with sterile saline should be introduced into the wound or lesion and removed without touching the adjacent tissues.

c. The sterile swab should be immediately put into the sterile test tube and the part of the swab handle touched by the fingers and hand in grasping should be broken off and discarded. Some commercials have plastic cap that covers the end of the swab handle and also serves as a cap for the test tube. Two cultures should be taken from each site so that one can be grown under aerobic conditions and the other under anaerobic conditions.

d. The cover of the test tube should then be screwed on tightly and the tube titled to saturate the swab with the transport media.

e. Sterile swabs in empty tubes. These are not to be used as they may cause death of organisms and alteration of flora [9].

8.2 Examination of exudates from inflammatory lesions: gingival pockets

Discharge from gingival abscess shows various types of pyogenic bacteria (*Staphylococcus*, *Streptococcus pyogenes* and pneumococcus species). Discharge from fistulae and gingival pockets may in addition show a large number of leukocytes. Appleton gives the following method of obtaining a specimen from the gingival pockets:

a. Isolate the area with sterile cotton rolls.

b. Stroke the gingival wall of the pocket to milk out the grosser quantity of microorganisms. With a sterile cotton pledget, wipe away the exudates.

c. Paint the gingival margin with tincture of iodine 1 part, acetone 1.5 parts and glycerin 0.5 part.

d. With a sterile flat platinum needle, collect material from the very depth of the pocket or draw a bit of the material into the capillary pipet.

e. Examine the specimen on a slide or else inoculate a number of deep test tubes of semi-liquid medium as ascitic fluid or ordinary nutrient agar plus a piece of fresh, sterile rabbit kidney tissue. This is satisfactory for the cultivation of many anaerobes [10, 11].

8.3 Bacteriologic tests of pulp canals

The technique for culture from pulp canals is:

a. Drying the canal with two or three sterile absorbent points.

b. Inserting a fresh sterile absorbent point and leaving it until the tip is moistened with the exudate (usually 1 min).

c. Removing the point with cotton pliers and, with one hand, opening the test tube of the medium held in the other hand.

d. Flaming the test tube lip, dropping the point into the tube, and plugging or covering. Make certain that the point is in the medium.

e. Incubating for 48 h.

f. If the medium is clear after the incubation, it is assumed that there is no growth of organism although a smear may be taken as a check. If the medium is cloudy or a precipitate is seen, assume that infection is still present. In questionable cases a second culture is taken [10, 11].

9. Blood cultures

These are used if bacteremia or septicemia is suspected. *Streptococci*, *Staphylococci* or *Pneumococci* may be found. In patients with multiple osteomyelitis, with extreme lesions in mandible, blood cultures showed that streptococcal septicemia was the cause. In chronic cases at least 15–30 cc. of blood should be taken for the test; in acute cases, 5 cc. is sufficient.

9.1 Examination of exudates for actinomycosis

In actinomycosis the discharge pressed out from the fistula contains the so-called sulfur granules. When soft, these granules can be pressed between two slides and examined without staining. The granules appear as rosette-like masses with dense centers and a network of mycelium. Bulbous clubs or rays extend from the periphery.

9.2 Examination for *Candida albicans*

Where thrush is suspected, moist preparations may be used, placing scrapings from the suspected lesion directly on a microscopic slide. A 10% solution of potassium hydroxide is added, and the slide is heated slightly and inspected under the microscope. The slide is examined for the branching mycelia and for spores of ***Candida albicans*** [11].

9.3 Examination of cystic fluid

Cysts contain a fluid or semi-fluid material, which for diagnostic purposes is aspirated by the means of glass syringe and hypodermic needle. The anesthetized place where the needle is to be inserted or the bone perforated with a sterilizing agent is prepared; the area with sterile gauze should be isolated. The cystic content is then aspirated and examined on a slide or cultured [10].

9.4 Transportation of diagnostic specimens

With the increasing specimen loads and collection centers now at the remotest parts of the country, transportation of the pathology specimen plays a crucial role in timely diagnosis. Thus specimen transport needs special care and attention to detail and appropriately filled laboratory requisition form guidelines that are usually issued by the national authorities, e.g., Infectious Diseases Society of America (IDSA) and the American Society for Microbiology (ASM) or Indian Council for Medical Research (ICMR) and the World Health Organization (WHO), are to be strictly followed.

For any hand-carried specimen that is transported over a short distance, the specimen needs to be placed upright in appropriate bottles with sufficient fixatives in appropriate racks. For long-distance cross country or different countries, the triple packing system has been advocated specially for infectious substances [12].

The triple packing system contains three layers as (1) primary container/ receptacle that has the specimen and is leak proof with a screw cap and (2) secondary container that is durable, waterproof and made of metal/plastic with a screw cap. It contains absorptive material, and details of the specimen are pasted on the outside of the container. (3) The outer packing or tertiary container is made of wood or card-box and withstands the transportation shocks. Dry ice is normally kept between the outer two containers with provision for carbon dioxide gas release vents. A biohazard label is a must [12].

9.5 Basic criteria for rejection of specimens

A laboratory should always consider strict rules on the basis of which an oral specimen could be rejected. This important decision must be taken with full conviction of doing the right thing to save time and laboratory resources. Such decision should be taken when the following criteria are not fulfilled:

1. Inappropriate test requests (incomplete, duplicate, missing or inconsistent information)

2. Errors in transport and handling (light exposure, delayed transport time or broken sample bottles)

3. Misidentification of specimen (unlabeled or mismatched)

4. Improper or wrong container

5. Insufficient specimen quantity for the quantity of preservative or insufficient quantity for the test requested transport media

6. Contamination of specimen

7. Incorrect storage

8. Hemolyzed sample [13]

10. Conclusions

Thus a continuous effort must be made in order to ensure proper collection and transportation of clinical specimens by all involved. A sound understanding of contemporary principles and practices of various methods of collection and transport of specimens is of critical importance to the clinician dealing with oral and maxillofacial infections.

Acknowledgements

The author K.S.S would like to thank her teachers Dr. Jyoti Chawda and Dr. Raksha Shah.

Conflict of interest

The authors declare no conflict of interest.

Author details

Krishna Sireesha Sundaragiri[1*], Soumya Makarla[2] and Bharat Sankhla[1]

1 Department of Oral Pathology, RUHS College of Dental Sciences (Government Dental College), Jaipur, Rajasthan, India

2 Department of Pathology and Microbiology, Krishnadevaraya College of Dental Sciences, Bengaluru, India

*Address all correspondence to: sksireesha@yahoo.co.in

References

[1] Mehrotra R, editor. Oral Cytology: A Concise Guide. New York: Springer-Verlag; 2013. DOI: 10.1007/978-1-4614-5221-8

[2] Mukherjee KL. Medical Laboratory Technology: A Procedure Manual for Routine Diagnostic Tests. Vols 1 and 2. 1st ed. New Delhi, India: McGraw Hill Education; 1988. pp. 486-564. Chapter 5

[3] Miloro M, Larsen P, Ghali GE, Waite PD. Peterson's Principles of Oral and Maxillofacial Surgery. 2nd ed. Hamilton: B.C. Decker Publications; 2004. Chapter 21

[4] Orel S, Sterrett GF. Orell & Sterrett's Fine Needle Aspiration Cytology. 5th ed. London: Churchill Livingstone; 2011

[5] Barnes L, editor. Surgical Pathology of the Head and Neck. 3rd ed. Vol. 1. USA: Informa Healthcare; 2008

[6] Vissink A, Wolff A, Veerman ECI. Chapter 4: Salivary diagnostics. In: Wong DT, editor. Saliva Collectors. Ames, IA: Wiley-Blackwell; 2008. p. 37

[7] Topizan RG, Goldberg MH, editors. Oral and Maxillofacial Infections. 3rd & 4th ed. Philadelphia: Saunders; 1993 and 2002

[8] Koneman EW, Allen SD, Janda WM, Schreckenberger PC, Winn WC. Color Atlas and Textbook of Diagnostic Microbiology. 5th ed. Philadelphia, United States: Lippincott Williams and Wilkins; 1997

[9] Thoma KT, Robinson HBG. Oral and dental diagnosis (with suggestions for treatment). In: Special Examinations for Dental and Oral Diseases. 5th ed. Philadelphia, London: WB Saunders; 1955

[10] Sabes WR. The Dentist and Clinical Laboratory Procedures. Mosby; 1979

[11] Molinari JA. Diagnostic modalities for infectious diseases. Dental Clinics of North America. 2003;**47**(4):605-621. DOI: 10.1016/j.cden.2003.08.001

[12] World Health Organization. Guidelines for the Safe Transport of Infectious Substances and Diagnostic Specimens. Division of Emerging and Other Communicable Diseases Surveillance and Control. 1997. Available from: https://www.who.int/csr/emc97_3.pdf

[13] Dikmen ZG, Pinar A, Akbiyik F. Specimen rejection in laboratory medicine: Necessary for patient safety? Biochemical Medicine. 2015;**25**(3):377-385

Chapter 4

Contemporary Overview of Blood Concentrates in Oral and Maxillacial Surgery

Onur Gönül, Ahmet Usame Çiçek, Murat Afat, Onur Atali and Faysal Uğurlu

Abstract

It has always been a target to shorten and improve the healing process in medical field. Platelets with cytokines and growth factors in their structure have great importance on wound healing. Features of platelets gave the clinicians the idea of using platelet concentrates to promote the healing process. For this reason, many platelet-derived biomaterials have been tried in the medical field over the years. When approaching today, platelet concentrates have been found to be used medically, especially with the use of platelet rich plasmas (PRPs) and then platelet rich fibrins (PRFs). In particular, several studies conducted in recent years have revaled different blood concentrates. This chapter summarizes the develoment over time, properties and usage areas of blood concentrates in dentistry.

Keywords: platelet rich fibrin, platelet rich plasma, sinus lifting, growth factor, graft, regeneration, oral and maxillofacial surgery

1. Introduction

Platelets are the smallest, colorless blood cells which paly a majör role in coagulation cascade and prevent excessive blood loss. Plateletsb diameters varies between 1-3 microns and they appear in a bright blue color under the microscope. Low platelet rate causes an increase in the tendency to bleed, and high platelet rate causes a clot (thrombosis) formation in the vein [1].

Platelets provide their functions with secretory granules in which there is a reservoir in its structure and freshly synthesized mediators. These granules consists ATP, ADP, serotonin, fibrinogen, plasminogen, platelet derived growth factor (PDGF), transforming growth factor beta (TGF-β), vascular endothelial growth factor (VEGF), epidermal growth factor (EGF), insulin like growth factor (IGF), etc. The growth factors have stimulating effect on wound healing by means of potential for matrix remodeling, cell proliferation and angiogenesis [2, 3].

Accordong to several researches, main task of platelets in the body is hemostasis and final clot formation in bleeding areas. In addition to their hemostatic duties, they are also effective in the tissue repair process due to the long term effects of these growth factors in theri structure [2, 3].

Platelets are counted among the potential cells of regenerative therapy. For the fact that they consist a large number of growth factors and are easy to obtain, has increased the interest in platelets. Tissue regeneration enginering is a field that many studies and attempts have been made about repairing a diseased tissue, regenerating or restoring a damaged tissue. Initially, studies have included allografts, xenografts, synthetic-based alloplasts, etc. However, most of these materials were observed to cause foreign body reaction in the body, which lead the studies to the human bodys's own tissues [4–7].

Ideas based on the use of human blood proteins as sources for regeneration arise from the idea that blood-derived proteins are a source of growth factors that can support angiogenesis and tissue growth for tissue regeneration. The healing process required for regeneration consists of hemostasis, inflammation, proliferation and maturation phases. Each phase requires its own specific proteins and cell types. However, since the non-human biomaterials used are avascular, the use of blood concentrates becomes more prominent [4–7].

As mentioned earlier, wound healing is a process that occurs as a result of hemostasis, inflammation, proliferation and maturation phases. Platelets are essential components that play an active role in the stages of hemostasis and fibrin formation, that is, in the early phases of the tissue regeneration process. Platelets secrete and contain some growth factors such as PDGF (Platelet derived growth factor), VEGF (Vascular endothelial growth factor), cytokines, etc., as well as angiogenetic factors that stimulate proliferation and activate the wound healing cells such as fibroblasts, neutrophils and mesenchymal stem cells [3, 8].

2. History of blood concentrates

The use of blood concentrates in medical field for various purposes is common for a long period of time. When we look at its historical background, the idea was used in the 1970s to be used for nerve tissue repair. The first use of platelet-rich plasma was reported in 1987 by Ferrari et al. during cardiac surgery and PRP was used to repair damaged cardiovascular tissues [9].

Looking at its use in dentistry, in the late 1990s, Whitman et al. suggested using PRP in oral surgical procedures, observing that PRP enhanced osteoprogenitor cells in bone graft and bone tissue. However, it is reported that depending on the use of bovine thrombin, coagulopathies and immune reactions can be observed [9, 10].

PRF is considered as the current platelet concentrate and has been used in oral and maxillofacial surgery since 2001. According to Choukroun et al. who first described PRFs in literature, PRFs have some advantages compared to PRPs, such as easier preparation and no chemical intervention to blood concentrates [11].

According to leukocyte and fibrin content, Verma et al. divided the platelet concentrates into 4 basic categories. They categorized platelet concentrates as P-PRP, L-PRP, P-PRF, and L-PRF [12].

Choukroun, the first person to report the use of PRF in 2001, described A-PRF, a new form of PRF, containing higher amounts of leukocytes in 2014. According to Choukroun, this new type of PRF has more potential than the original PRF [13].

3. Classification of blood concentrates

The story of blood concentrates is usually examined in 2 parts/generations. Here we see the PRPs first, and the PRFs as the second generation. Classification is simply done as follows:

- P-PRP (1. GENERATION)
- L-PRP (1. GENERATION)
- P-PRF (2. GENERATION)
- L-PRF (2. GENERATION)
- I-PRF (2. GENERATION)
- A-PRF (2. GENERATION)
- T-PRF (2 GENERATION)

4. Preparation procedures and clinical features of PRPs

Basically, the aim of the formation of blood concentrates is to achieve higher platelet density and high level of growth hormones. PRPs are also tried to be prepared for this purpose. PRPs are basically condensed plasma with a higher platelet concentration than the normal state of the blood. PRPs show high platelet and growth factor levels compared to normal blood. It has been determined that PRPs have positive effects on periodontal cells, osteoblasts, etc. after their use [9, 14–18].

Despite their benefits, PRPs have some disadvantages. They are obtained in a multi-stage and long process, difficult to handle and expensive to obtain. PRPs usually have two basic centrifuge steps. Ethylenediaminetetraacetic acid (EDTA) or citric acid can be used in the first slow centrifuge step. Then comes the second centrifuge step, which is applied faster. At this stage, additional substances such as calcium chloride or/and bovine thrombin can be used. These additives, in fact, cause blood concentrates, which are of interest as being autologous, to loose their full autologous feature. In addition, foreign substances -especially bovine thrombin-which are included in the PRPs, increase the potential of PRPs to create a foreign body reaction. Accordingly, the natural inflammatory process of the body can be disrupted. In addition, artificial clotting is provided while obtaining PRP. Accordingly, the fibrin matrix structure formed is different from the structure obtained naturally. The fibrin matrix structure obtained in this way is more rigid. Due to this rigid structure, it does not release the growth factors in the PRP in a controlled and long term and releases all at once. Also bovine thrombin can cause the risk of coagulopathy as well as foreign body reaction. It also increases the cost of preparing PRPs with special kits and spending a lot of time. PRPs are often used by mixing with grafts due to the disadvantage of their liquid structures during use [9, 14–18].

5. Preparation procedures and clinical features of PRFs

Despite the high platelet and growth factor ratios provided by PRPs, the observed negativities pushed clinicians to new researches. As a result, PRFs, which are the second generation blood concentrates and have the advantages of being prepared more quickly, have emerged. PRFs appeared mainly as blood concentrates created without using additive anticoagulants. A single, high-speed return is achieved in obtaining the PRF. In the most basic centrifuge method that provides the PRFs, single centrifugation is performed for 12 minutes at 2700-3000 rpm per minute [4, 19–23].

In this way, three layers are obtained:

- Protein Poor Plasma (PPP)
- Platelet Rich Fibrin (PRF)
- Red Blood Cells (RBC)

As studies based on PRF progressed, it was understood that the amount of leukocytes in the content had an important effect on ideal wound healing. This is the reason why leukocyte content is also taken into account in the classification of PRFs. The presence of leukocytes has been found to be effective in obtaining clinical results ideally and achieving lower infection rates. PRFs are structures that contain important cells for healing process of the body, but it is also important that they form a three-dimensional matrix and contain significant growth factors [4, 12, 19–23].

PRFs, of course, did not remain as they first appeared, but were developed in time. PRFs with different contents were obtained by applying different centrifuge methods. The first obtained P-PRF consisted of a solid fibrin matrix structure and did not contain leukocytes. Later, L-PRF appeared, known as leukocyte and platelet-rich fibrin. The A-PRFs were produced by Choukroun, the first revealer of PRFs. This type of PRF has a better handling than other types of PRFs. It is obtained by low speed centrifuge. 14-minute centrifuge process at 1500 rpm is required for the A-PRF acquisition. A-PRFs are blood concentrates containing high amounts of leukocytes. In addition, I-PRFs, an injectable form of PRFs, have emerged. I-PRFs are a type of PRF that can also contain stem cells. To obtain it, centrifuge should be applied for 3-4 minutes at 800 rpm. Another type of PRF is T-PRF. The main difference is that

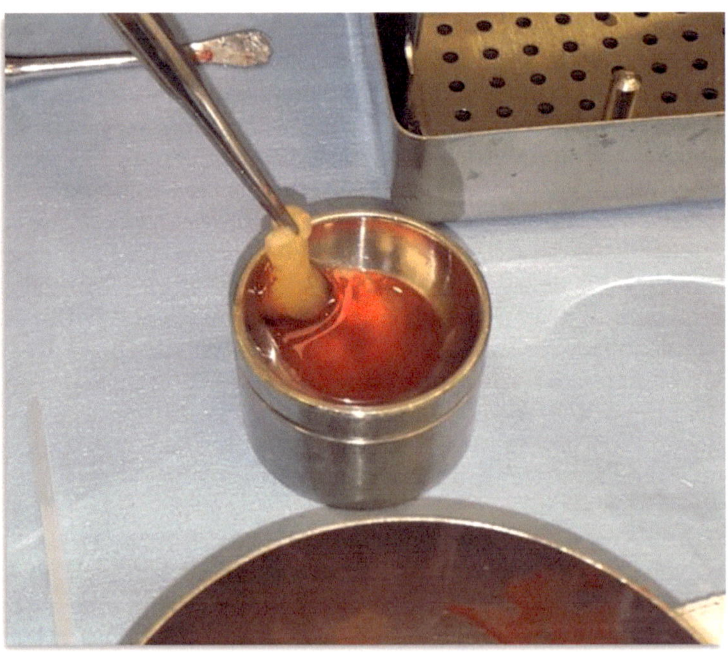

Figure 1.
PRF clot just after centrifuge.

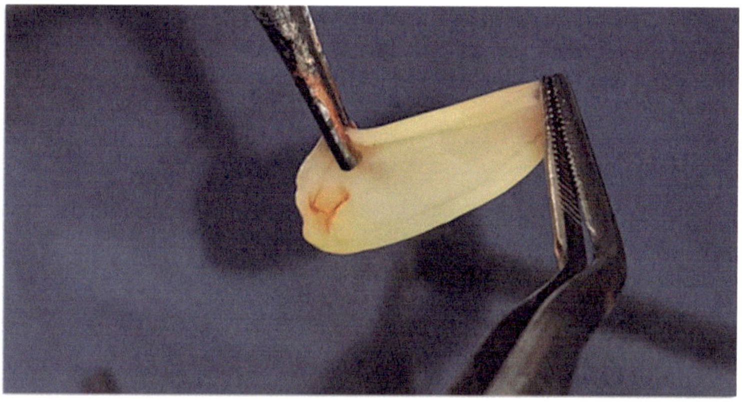

Figure 2.
PRF membrane after pressing PRF clot between two sterile surfaces.

the tubes are made of titanium. According to some studies fibrin matrix obtained in this method is considered to be more successful (**Figures 1** and **2**) [4, 12, 19–23].

PRFs have been of great interest and improved platelet concentrates for many years. The reason for this is of course their advantages. Unlike the PRPs we mentioned earlier, PRFs are produced completely autogenously. There is no need for extra biochemical interventions. It has an easy application procedure. The method is inexpensive since there is no kit requirement or extra process requirement mentioned in PRPs. Since there is no substance added from the outside, fibrinogen turns into fibrin thanks to the thrombin that is found in the blood spontaneously. In this way, the mechanism operates slowly and in accordance with its natural state. The fibrin thus formed is also a close to nature fibrin. Cell migration and proliferation increased compared to PRP. There are studies showing that it positively affects osteoblast activity. Also, when compared with PRP, it is seen that PRFs have higher fibrin content [4, 19–23].

In addition to the many advantageous features described, PRFs also have some disadvantages. Blood is required to be applied. This situation creates anxiety in patients or increases the tendency to refuse treatment. When it is desired to obtain high amounts of PRF, serious blood intake is needed. There is a need for a glass-coated tube to perform the process [19–23].

6. Application fields in dentistry

PRFs have been used in many fields of medicine and dentistry since its occurrence. It is used in general medicine especially in orthopedic field and for the healing of open wounds and ulcers. In dentistry, it is used in endodontics, periodontology and oral and maxillofacial surgery. Main fields of clinical usage are given below [4, 19–23].

ENDODONTICS:

- Can be used for pulp regeneration
- It can be used for apex formation procedures.
- It can be used in the treatment of periapical cysts.

- Can be used as a pulp capping material.

PERIODONTOLOGY:

- It is used to treat intrabony defects.
- It is used to stimulate wound healing after periodontal surgery.
- For coverage of open root surfaces

ORAL and MAXILLOFACIAL SURGERY:

- It is used to protect the socket.
- It is used to prevent alveolitis.
- It is used to ensure the ideal healing of the area after apical surgery.
- It is applied to the peri-implant region to support osseointegration.
- It is used in grafting procedures in bone deficiencies.
- Can be used with or without grafts in sinus lifting procedures.
- It can be used to accelerate recovery after surgery for osteonecrosis.
- It can be used as matrix in biomaterial applications.

7. Biological view of PRFs

Understanding the biological properties of PRFs depends on having information about the content. Also, it is important to know the wound healing process to understand the effects of PRF. The healing of wounds is a process that starts with the hemostasis mechanism and continues with a series of events. The effect of PRFs depends on some key features. The first is the presence of the fibrin matrix. In this way, the fibrin matrix acts as a scaffolding where the cells providing the construction events migrate. The second is the fibrin matrix and the cells in it; secrete chemotactic proteins, cytokines and growth factors. The third is that the fibrin matrix and its factors induce vascular structure formation [4].

The effects of PRFs come from the elements in it. Its structure consists of fibrin matrix and cellular elements. The most important cell in its structure as a cellular element is of course platelets. In addition, its structure includes leukocytes, neutrophils, monocytes and mesenchymal stem cells. Growth factors, which are considered as the most important content of PRFs, are secreted by other cellular elements, especially platelets. The secretion of growth factors and their functions are very important for the functions of PRFs [4].

We know that PRFs provide secretion of many growth factors. These factors and effects are given below;

- TGF-β1: This molecule is an important inflammation regulator. It is also a very strong fibrosis agent. Its most important tasks are tissue repair, immune modulation and extracellular matrix synthesis. In addition, TGF-β1 plays an important role in collagen production. TGF-β1 also plays a role in restoring epithelialization and connective tissue healing. Transforming growth factor beta is also a critical mediator for bone formation. It stimulates the chemotaxis, cleavage and accumulation of osteoblasts [4, 24–26].

- PDGF: This growth factor known as platelet derived growth factor is important for the proliferation, migration and survival of mesenchymal cells. This growth factor also enables extracellular matrix production to occur during tissue healing. He is also involved in collagen production-demolition mechanisms. PDGF is also a mitogen factor for osteoblast and fibroblast cells [4, 24–26].

- EGF: It stands for epidermal growth factor. The receptors of this factor are expressed in the majority of human cells, including cells that are important in wound healing stages. EGF stimulates the division of mesenchymal stem cells. It also provides chemotaxis in endothelial cells [4, 24–26].

- VEGF: Vascular endothelial growth factor is most commonly secreted by platelets and macrophages. This growth factor is the most active growth factor for vascular regeneration. It provides angiogenesis and the formation of new blood vessels. In this way, blood flow and thus nutrition increase in injured tissues [4, 24–26].

- IGF: Insulin-like growth factor is released when platelets are activated. It induces the differentiation and division of mesenchymal stem cells. IGF is also one of the mediators involved in the regulation of the programmed cell death process. Besides, IGF stimulates proliferation and differentiation in many cells of the body. IGF is also involved in bone matrix formation and replication of osteoblasts [4, 24–26].

8. Clinical applications in maxillofacial surgery

8.1 Sinus lifting

The high healing potential and ingredients of the PRFs have brought to mind the ideas of both increasing the success and shortening the healing time by using them in sinus lifting procedures. Based on these ideas, PRFs were used in sinus lifting procedures, firstly mixed with grafts and then without using grafts. In studies conducted, it has been observed that even though there are no large differences in the amount of bone tissue obtained as a result of mixing graft materials and PRFs, it accelerates the maturation and the wound healing period. In addition, using PRFs mixed with graft materials makes the manipulation of the graft material quite easy. In addition, when PRF membranes are used in sinus lifting procedures instead of other membranes, PRF membranes have been found to be an inexpensive, easy-to-manipulate membrane, so they can be used to close lateral sinus Windows (**Figure 3**). When used for closing the lateral sinus window, it speeds up the healing process and provides good protection for the Schneiderian membrane (**Figure 4**). In cases where the Schneiderian membrane is perforated, PRF membranes are used to make a healing barrier for the perforation zone [27–31].

Although PRFs have the expectation of controlling tissue inflammation with their special biological properties and providing good vascularization in bone tissue, the studies conducted have not yet shown a common understanding of their effects in the literature [27–32].

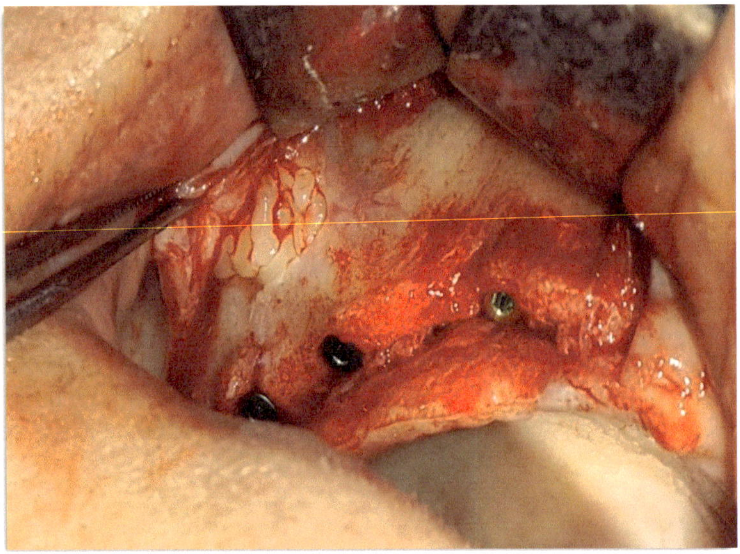

Figure 3.
Application of PRF as a bulk matrix for sinus lifting.

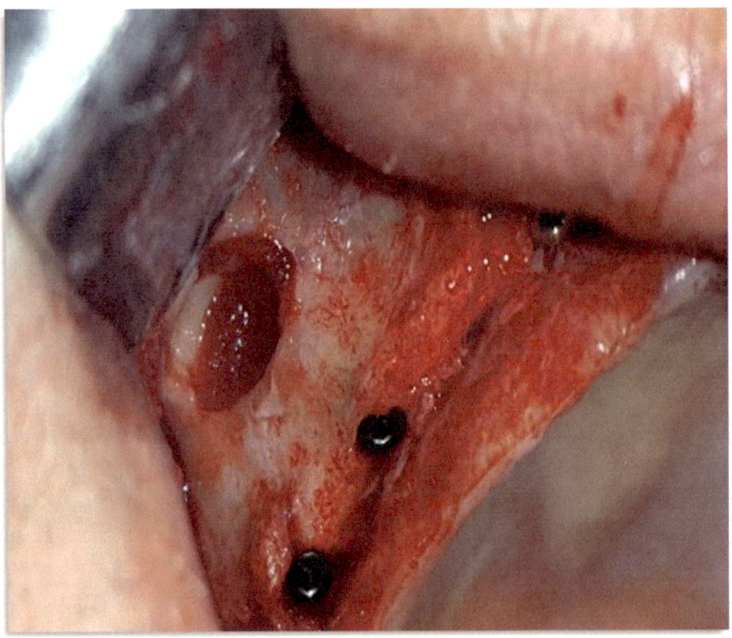

Figure 4.
Application of PRF as a membrane on sinus membrane.

8.2 Alveolar socket preservation

Studies on PRF consider that the use of PRF accelerates epithelialization and vascularization so that wound healing takes place effectively and quickly. However, operations such as tooth extractions and cyst enucleations lead to bone defects after healing process. These defect areas creates esthetic and functional deficiency problems for patients. By using PRFs on healing processes, it has been thought that healing of intra-bony sockets in the alveolar area can be accelerated and bone defect formation can be reduced (**Figure 5**) [32–34].

There are studies that believe that PRFs inserted into the sockets do not make a significant difference in preventing complications in the post-operative period, as some studies show that there is a significant decrease in the frequency of occurrence of alveolar osteitis and bone loss in patients, especially after the 3rd molar surgery. In addition, it is seen that there is no definite opinion about bone gain and remodeling in the literature. However, it is possible to say that the use of PRF improves the patient experience by reducing the frequency of complications such as pain and swelling in the post-operative period. However, its cost is very low, making it attractive to use for post-operative socket protection [34–37].

8.3 Alveolar ridge augmentations

The use of PRF draws attention in augmentation procedures in many fields. PRFs are used for more than one purpose in guided bone regeneration (GBR). PRFs can be used as membranes or preferred to speed up the wound healing process. Studies showed that PRF membranes are successful in closing bone defects. However, the use of PRFs as a barrier membrane in GBR processes alone creates a question. In addition, injecting PRFs into the region in liquid form or placing PRF membranes around the collagen membranes used can stimulate and accelerate soft tissue healing in the region (**Figure 6**). Besides, it can stimulate bone tissue healing. The use of PRF has the potential to increase bone vascularization in areas where GBR is performed. Also, mixing of PRFs with grafts increases the stability and manipulation potential of the grafts in augmentations (**Figures 7–9**) [38–41].

8.4 Implants and PRF

Marginal bone loss may occur following implantation. In order to repair or stop these bone losses, many studies have been performed over the years and different methods have been explained. The clinicians, who thought that marginal bone loss around the implant was completely caused by soft tissue quality and health, thought that PRFs, which are considered to be a very successful material when used in soft tissue augmentation, will completely stop marginal bone loss. There are also studies reporting that the use of PRF in defects around implants, the use of PRFs in flap operations and grafting procedures, yields better results than standard protocols. However, there are no definitive results in the literature regarding the effect of PRF use on hard tissue augmentation and it is stated that more studies are needed [42, 43].

Another area in which PRFs are used in relation to dental implants is their impact on implant stability. In studies conducted on this subject, the stability of the implants was measured by making early resonance frequency analyzes. In the

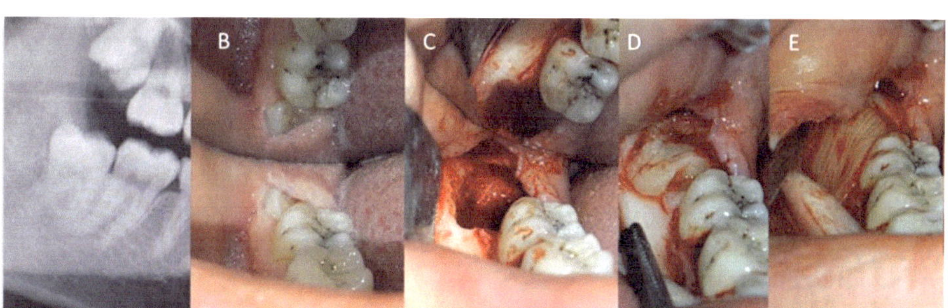

Figure 5.
Using PRF in the extraction socket.

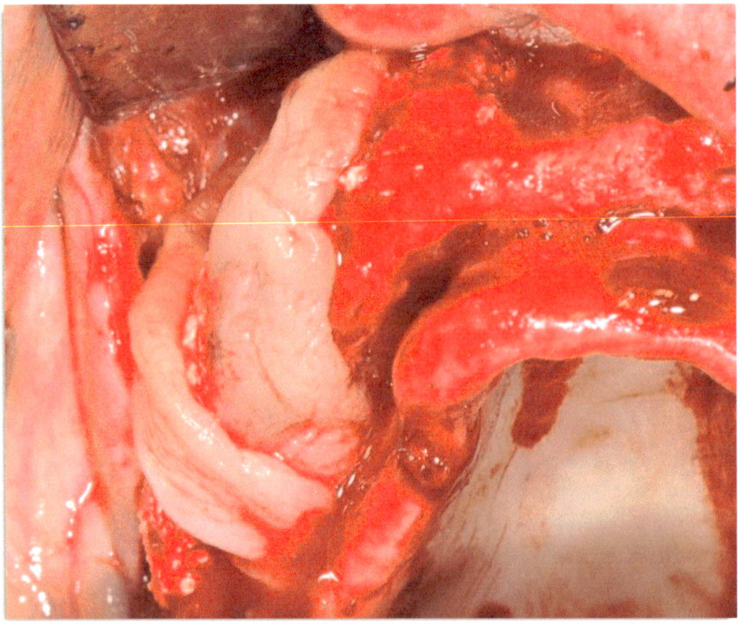

Figure 6.
PRF membranes on the particulated xenografts grafts.

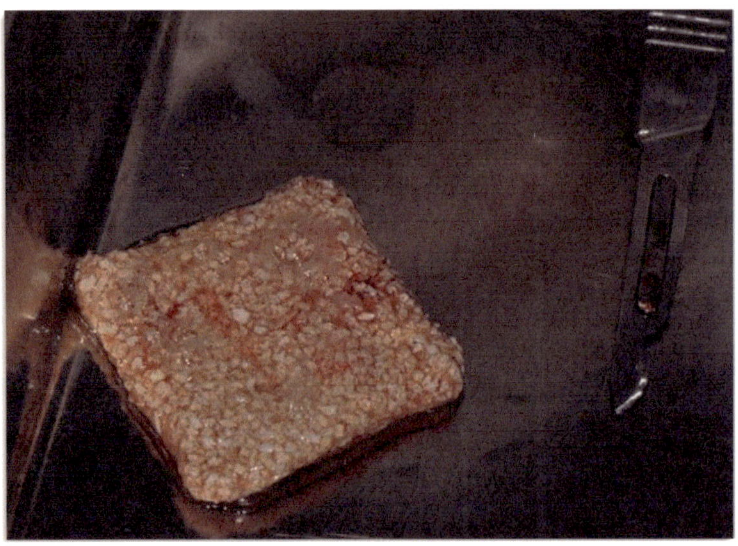

Figure 7.
PRF with bone graft.

studies conducted, it is generally believed that the use of PRF increases the ISQ values of the implants in the early healing period [44–46].

Thanks to the cytokines it contains, it can be used to control inflammation in the inflammatory conditions around the implant as well as in the sockets. Besides, PRFs can be useful in increasing gingival quality and peri-implant periodontal tissue regeneration processes [44–46].

PRFs can be useful in immediate implantation situations where implantation will be performed immediately after extraction. The most important reason for this

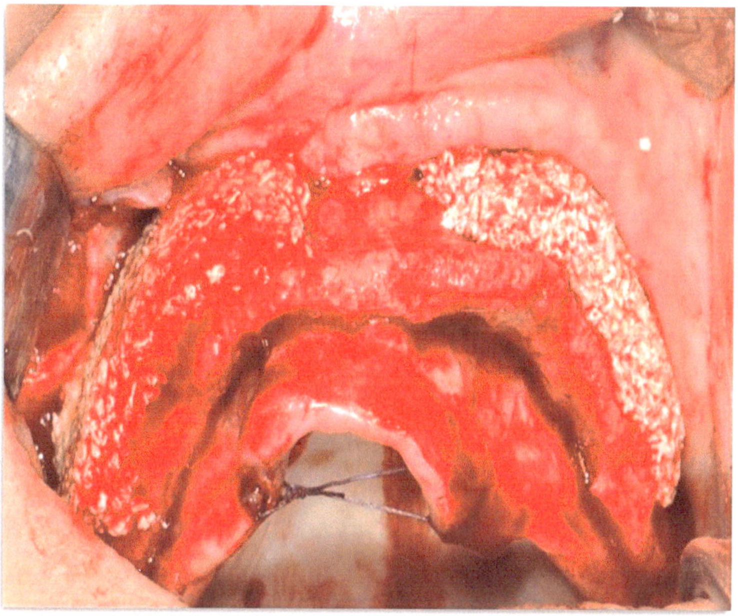

Figure 8.
Alveolar ridge augmentation.

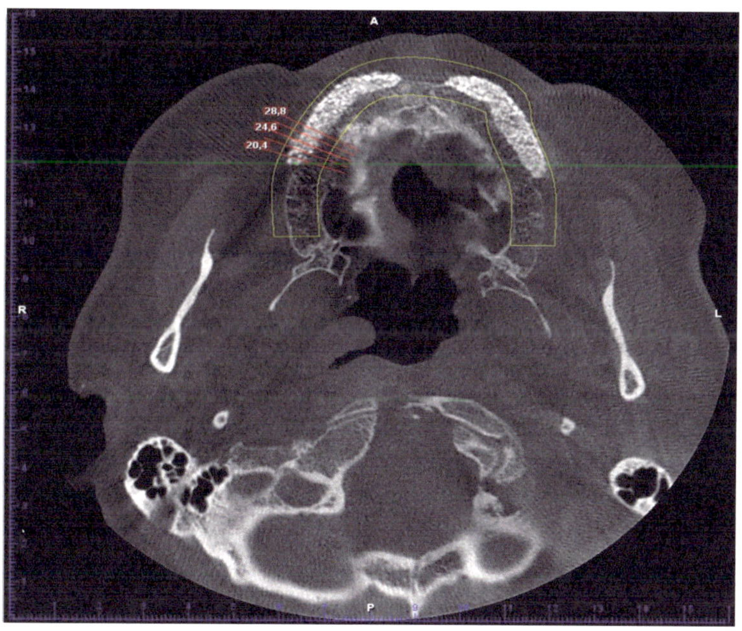

Figure 9.
Grafted area on the CBCCT after 6 months of application.

are the growth factors and cytokines. Thanks to these substances, it will create a high healing potential. In addition, the gaps between the implant and the bone wall can be filled using PRF in immediate implantations. This can only be done by using PRF or by mixing PRF and bone graft materials. However, in cases using collagen membranes, the potential for soft tissue healing can be increased by using PRF (**Figures 10–13**) [47, 48].

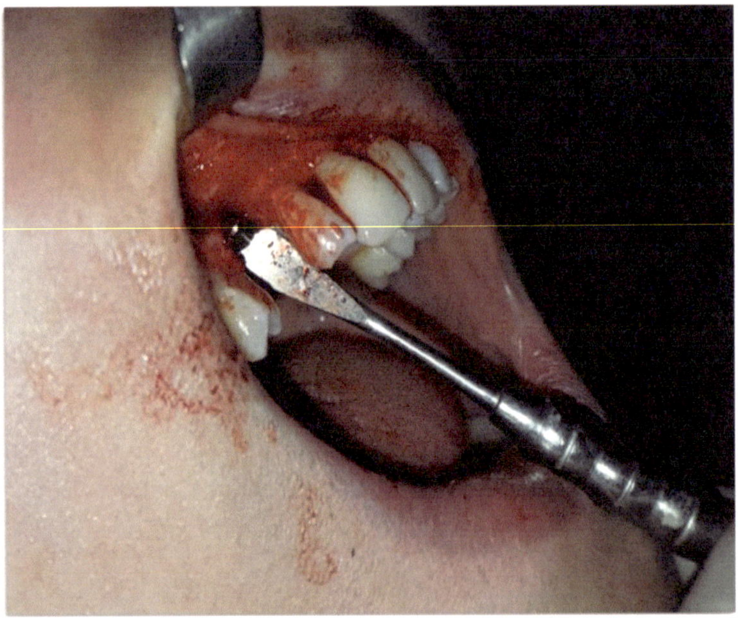

Figure 10.
Deficient bone around implant.

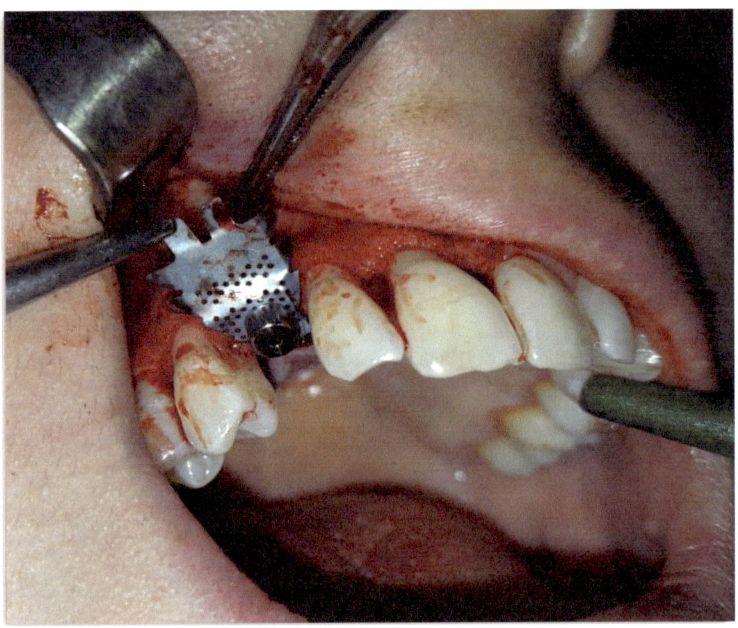

Figure 11.
Titanium mesh application for GBR.

8.5 PRF applications in other fields oral and maxillofacial surgery

In oral surgery practice, oroantral fistulas may occur due to the morphology of the region or due to iatrogenic reasons in the attempts made in the posterior maxilla. Oroantral fistula formation can often occur due to tooth extractions from the region, after cyst excisions or in relation to implant surgery. In the process of

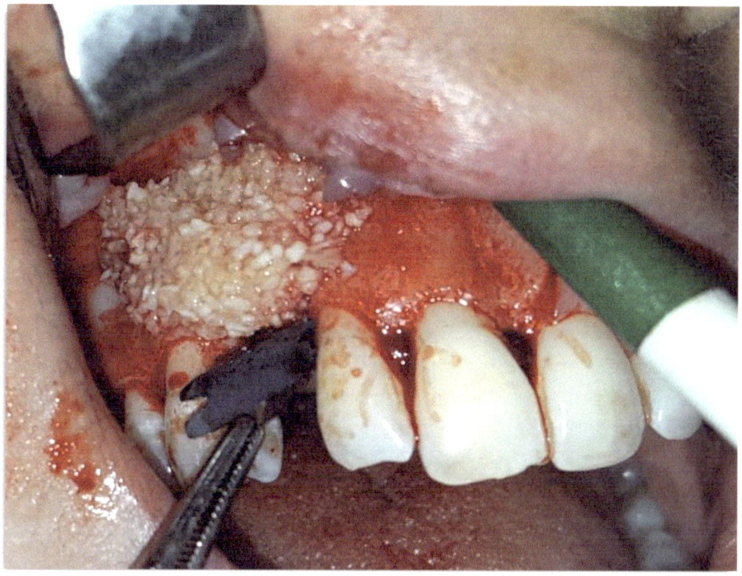

Figure 12.
Application of graft material.

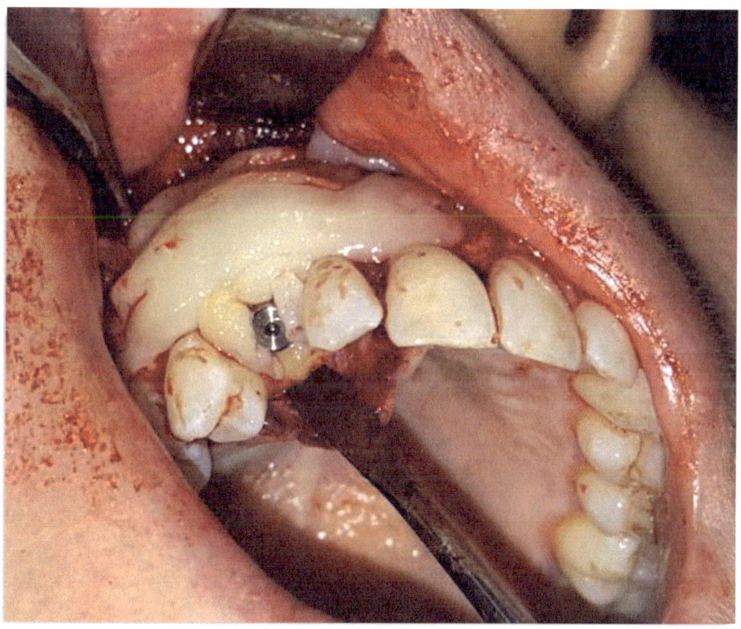

Figure 13.
PRF insertion over Ti-mesh membrane.

closing these fistulas, generally shifted flap techniques are used. However, in recent years, PRF has been used to close these defects. After the region is removed from infected tissues as in other techniques, PRF is applied to the area as thin membranes. In this way, it is not necessary to use outsourced material or use techniques that create serious donor site morbidity [49–51].

Intraoral osteonecrosis scenarios appear due to various medical conditions, especially bisphosphonate group drugs. Generally, some studies in recent years have suggested the use of PRF in osteonecrosis cases, which is tried to be treated in various ways such as curettage, hyperbaric oxygen therapy, laser stimulations. It has been reported that PRF can act as a barrier membrane and accelerate soft tissue healing around the necrotic areas [52, 53].

PRFs can be used in the surgery of alveolar clefts apart from many other areas mentioned. In addition, it can be used to stimulate healing in patients who have or are likely to experience a healing problem due to medical problems [54].

9. PRF for endodontics

As a result of recent studies, regenerative endodontic therapies have begun to take their place among endodontics procedures. Regenerative procedures are mainly aimed at making the pulp functional by stimulating the pulp tissue that loses its function and cells with the potential for change in it [55, 56].

In the light of the studies, it was seen that PRFs can be used for regeneration in endodontics. For this purpose, in endodontics, PRF can be used for apex closure procedures and for revascularization procedures [55, 56].

In some of the studies conducted, PRF was used with MTA to manage the formation of apex. As a result, it was observed that beneficial results were obtained by using two materials together. The reason for the promising results obtained by using two materials together is that they work synergistically when they are together and thus stem cell and odontoblast stimulation is considered to be more successful [55–59].

Another area regarding the use of PRFs in endodontics is revascularization procedures. It is thought that PRFs can be used as scaffold material for regeneration of necrotic pulp and it is an ideal material as scaffold. The reason for this is, of course, the high amount of growth factors that PRF contains. Thus, it is a very successful skeleton for regeneration. In addition, the coronal pulp removed in regenerative pulpotomy procedures can be replaced with PRF to cover the underlying live pulp. Then it is covered with mineral trioxide aggregate (MTA). PRFs are also included in the apical surgery in the endodontic field. In this field, there are authors who say that the PRFs are successful, as well as the authors who say that the PRFs did not make a significant change. PRFs are thought to be mixed with MTA to create root end barrier. In order to fill the bone cavities formed after apical surgery, good results can be obtained by mixing the bone grafts and PRF [55–59].

10. Using PRFs in periodontology

In the field of periodontology, PRFs are used in the treatment of gingival recessions, intra-bone defects, furcation defects, wound healing of hard and soft tissues, and regeneration of all periodontium tissues. Growth factors used in the periodontium tissues achieve their therapeutic and regenerating properties of tissues by providing differentiation and proliferation inducing effects such as angiogenesis, cementogenesis, differentiation of osteoblasts, anabolic bone formation, etc. Compared with traditional periodontal treatments, it is seen that PRF systems provide very useful results thanks to these properties [60–62].

In addition to periodontal flap applications in teeth with intra-bone defects, successful results are obtained by providing regeneration in hard and soft tissues in the region related to PRF applications. With the use of PRF in intra-bone defects, a decrease in pocket depth scores, an increase in clinical attachment level, and an increase in bone filling of the region are observed, and significant advantages are observed as a result of use alone or in combination with other biomaterials [63, 64].

As with intra-bone defects, PRF applications in furcation defects provide successful results with applications combined with traditional periodontal flap operations. Studies showed that the coronally advanced flap procedure gives more successful results when applied in combination with free connective tissue graft or PRF. Therefore; PRF applications are seen as an alternative to free tissue grafts in periodontal treatments [63, 64].

The use of PRF has been shown to have successful results in patients with aggressive periodontitis. As a result of the combined applications of PRF systems with traditional periodontal surgery, an increase in the level of attachment, decrease in pocket depth and long-term follow-up bone regeneration can be observed in the teeth with aggressive periodontitis [65].

When it comes to gingival recessions, coronally advanced flap procedure with subepithelial connective tissue are among the first periodontal treatments that come to mind. With the widespread use of PRF, the use of PRF instead of subepithelial connective tissue graft is still an area in which studies are ongoing. Compared to the subepithelial connective tissue, it does not create a donor site wound, healing process and preventing patient discomfort during this process are the most important advantages of PRF applications in this area [66, 67].

Another use of PRF membranes in periodontology is that it can be used as a palatal wound bandage or protective membrane after placement of connective tissue grafts. Studies show that it is an effective method to protect the newly formed wound area in palatina and to increase patient comfort by accelerating wound healing in the area [68, 69].

PRF applications are among the most up-to-date and promising areas of periodontology due to their versatile nature. PRFs can be applied alone to the defect surfaces, as well as combined with graft materials or can serve as a thin membrane in regenerative treatments. In addition to these features, they have the feature of being an alternative to connective tissue grafts, thanks to their cellular content, when appropriate. In addition to the aforementioned areas of use, they can function as wound plugs and provide graft stabilization. Considering all these, with its low cost and biological features, PRF applications are effective in many areas in periodontology [63, 64].

11. Conclusion

In many studies, successful results have been obtained from PRFs. It can be said that the most important reason for PRFs success is the growth factors in its own structure. The accelerator and strengthening effect of wound healing is quite obvious with their effect. Besides, it is seen that PRFs have positive effects in regeneration and augmentation procedures. Although more studies are needed on the use of PRFs in some specific areas, PRFs are used quite frequently. In the future, their use seems to increase in all fields of dentistry especially in oral and maxillofacial surgery.

Conflict of interest

The authors declare no conflict of interest.

Author details

Onur Gönül[1]*, Ahmet Usame Çiçek[1], Murat Afat[2], Onur Atali[1] and Faysal Uğurlu[1]

1 Department of Oral and Maxillofacial Surgery, Faculty of Dentistry, Marmara University, Istanbul, Turkey

2 Private Practice, İstanbul, Turkey

*Address all correspondence to: onurgonul@yahoo.com

References

[1] Koçyiğit İD, Tunali M, Özdemir H, Kartal Y, Süer BT. İkinci nesil trombosit konsantrasyonunun klinik uygulamalari. Cumhuriyet Dental Journal 2012;15(3):279-87.

[2] Wachowicz B, Morel A, Miller E, Saluk J. The physiology of blood platelets and changes of their biological activities in multiple sclerosis. Acta Neurobiol Exp 2016;76:269-81.

[3] Toker H, Alpan AL, Hocaoglu TP. Management of Mandibular Osteomyelitis Combined with Platelet Rich Fibrin (PRF) and Ozone. Cumhuriyet Dental Journal 2016;19(3):189-96.

[4] Kobayashi E, Fluckiger L, Fujioka-Kobayashi M, Sawada K, Sculean A, Schaller B, et al. Comparative release of growth factors from PRP, PRF, and advanced-PRF. Clinical oral investigations. 2016.

[5] Lucarelli E, Beretta R, Dozza B, Tazzari PL, O'Connel SM, Ricci F, et al. A recently developed bifacial platelet-rich fibrin matrix. European cells & materials. 2010; 20:13-23.

[6] Saluja H, Dehane V, Mahindra U. Platelet Rich fibrin: A second generation platelet concentrate and a new friend of oral and maxillofacial surgeons. Annals of maxillofacial surgery. 2011;1(1):53-7.

[7] Choukroun J, Adda F, Schoeffler C, Vervelle A. Une opportunit'e en paro-implantologie: le PRF. Implantodontie. 2001;42(55):e62.

[8] Aroca S, Keglevich T, Barbieri B, Gera I, Etienne D. Clinical evaluation of a modified coronally advanced flap alone or in combination with a platelet-rich fibrin membrane for the treatment of adjacent multiple gingival recessions: a 6-month study. Journal of periodontology 2009;80(2):244-52.

[9] Marx RE, Carlson ER, Eichstaedt RM, Schimmele SR, Strauss JE, Georgeff KR. Platelet-rich plasma: growth factor enhancement for bone grafts. Oral Surgery, Oral Medicine, Oral Pathology, Oral Radiology, and Endodontology 1998;85(6):638-46.

[10] Whitman DH, Berry RL, Green DM. Platelet gel: an autologous alternative to fibrin glue with applications in oral and maxillofacial surgery. Journal of oral and maxillofacial surgery. 1997;55(11):1294-9.

[11] Choukroun J, Adda F, Schoeffler C, Vervelle A. Une opportunité en paro-implantologie: le PRF. Implantodontie. 2000;42:55-62.

[12] Ehrenfest DMD, Rasmusson L, Albrektsson T. Classification of platelet concentrates: from pure platelet-rich plasma (P-PRP) to leucocyteand platelet-rich fibrin (L-PRF). Trends in biotechnology 2009;27(3):158-67.

[13] Choukroun J. Advanced PRF, &i-PRF: platelet concentrates or blood concentrates. J Periodont Med Clin Practice 2014;1:3.

[14] Plachokova AS, Nikolidakis D, Mulder J, Jansen JA, Creugers NH. Effect of platelet-rich plasma on bone regeneration in dentistry: a systematic review. Clin Oral Implants Res 2008;19(6):539-45. 19. Pietrzak WS, Eppley BL. Platelet rich plasma: biology and new technology. J Craniofac Surg 2005;16(6):1043-54.

[15] Pallua N, Wolter T, Markowicz M. Plateletrich plasma in burns. Burns 2010;36(1):4-8.

[16] Simon D, Manuel S, Geetha V, Naik BR. Potential for osseous regeneration of plateletrich plasma comparative study in mandibular

third molar sockets. Indian J Dent Res 2004;15(4):133-6.

[17] Everts PA, Brown Mahoney C, Hoffmann JJ, Schönberger JP, Box HA, Van Zundert A, Knape JT. Platelet-rich plasma preparation using three devices: implications for platelet activation and platelet growth factor release. Growth factors 2006;24(3):165-71.

[18] Jo CH, Roh YH, Kim JE, Shin S, Yoon KS. Optimizing platelet-rich plasma gel formation by varying time and gravitational forces during centrifugation. Journal of Oral Implantology 2013;39(5):525-32.

[19] Saluja H, Dehane V, Mahindra U. PlateletRich fibrin: A second generation platelet concentrate and a new friend of oral and maxillofacial surgeons. Annals of maxillofacial surgery 2011;1(1):53.

[20] Dohan DM, Choukroun J, Diss A, Dohan SL, Dohan AJ, Mouhyi J, Gogly B. Plateletrich fibrin (PRF): a second-generation platelet concentrate. Part II: platelet-related biologic features. Oral Surg Oral Med Oral Pathol Oral Radiol Endod 2006;101(3):e45-50.

[21] Castro AB, Meschi N, Temmerman A, Pinto N, Lambrechts P, Teughels W, Quirynen M. Regenerative potential of leucocyte- and platelet-rich fibrin. Part A: intra-bony defects, furcation defects and periodontal plastic surgery. A systematic review and metaanalysis. J Clin Periodontol 2017;44(1):67-82.

[22] Carroll R, Arnoczky S, Graham S, O'Connell S. Characterization of autologous growth factors in Cascade platelet rich fibrin matrix (PRFM). Edison, NJ: Musculoskeletal Transplant Foundation 2005.

[23] Verma UP, Yadav RK, Dixit M, Gupta A. Platelet-rich Fibrin: A Paradigm in Periodontal Therapy - A Systematic Review. J Int Soc Prev Community Dent 2017;7(5):227-33.

[24] Gurtner GC, Werner S, Barrandon Y, Longaker MT. Wound repair and regeneration. Nature. 2008; 453(7193):314-21.

[25] Amaranath J, Das N, Gupta R, Gupta I. Platelet-Rich Fibrin - A Biofuel for Periodontal and Tissue Regeneration: A Review Article. Rama Univ J Dent Sci. 2017; 4(2):14-22.

[26] Choukroun J, Diss A, Simonpieri A, Girard MO, Schoeffler C, Dohan AJ et al. Platelet-rich fibrin (PRF): a secondgeneration platelet concentrate, Part IV: clinical effects on tissue healing. Oral Surg Oral M

[27] Simonpieri A, Choukroun J, Del Corso M, Sammartino G, Dohan Ehrenfest DM. Simultaneous sinus-lift and implantation using microthreaded implants and leukocyte- and platelet-rich fibrin as sole grafting material: a six-year experience. Implant Dent. 2011;20:2-12.

[28] Mazor Z, Horowitz RA, Del Corso M, Prasad HS, Rohrer MD, Dohan Ehrenfest DM. Sinus floor augmentation with simultaneous implant placement using Choukroun's platelet-rich fibrin as the sole grafting material: a radiologic and histologic study at 6 months. J Periodontol. 2009;80:2056-2064.

[29] Toffler M, Toscano N, Holtzclaw D, Corso MD, Dohan Ehrenfest DM. Introducing Choukroun's platelet rich fibrin (PRF) to the reconstructive surgery milieu. J Implant Clin Adv Dent. 2009;1:21-30.

[30] Choukroun J, Diss A, Simonpieri A, Girard MO, Schoeffler C, Dohan SL, Dohan AJ, Mouhyi J, Dohan DM. Platelet-rich fibrin (PRF): a second-generation platelet concentrate. Part V:

histologic evaluations of PRF effects on bone allograft maturation in sinus lift. Oral Surg Oral Med Oral Pathol Oral Radiol Endod. 2006;101:299-303.

[31] Zhang Y, Tangl S, Huber CD, et al. Effects of Choukroun's platelet-rich fibrin on bone regeneration incombination with deproteinized bovine bone mineral in maxillary sinus augmentation: A histological and histomorphometric study. Journal of Cranio-Maxillo-Facial Surgery.2012;40:321-328

[32] Del Corso, M., Vervelle, A., Simonpieri, A., Jimbo, R., Inchingolo, F., Sammartino, G., & M Dohan Ehrenfest, D. (2012). Current knowledge and perspectives for the use of platelet-rich plasma (PRP) and platelet-rich fibrin (PRF) in oral and maxillofacial surgery part 1: Periodontal and dentoalveolar surgery. Current Pharmaceutical Biotechnology, 13(7), 1207-1230.

[33] Del Fabbro M, Bucchi C, Lolato A, et al. Autologous platelet concentrates to improve post extraction outcomes. Journal of Oral and Maxillofacial Surgery. 2017;75:1601-1615

[34] Moraschini V, Barboza ESP. Effect of autologous platelet concentrates for alveolar socket preservation: A systematic review. International Journal of Oral and Maxillofacial Surgery. 2015;44:632-641

[35] Nanditha S, Balamanikandasrinivasan C, Senthilkumar M, et al. Appraising the diverse facets of platelet rich fibrin in surgery through a systematic review. International Journal of Surgery. 2017;46:186-194

[36] Becker W, Urist M, Becker BE, et al. Clinical and histologic observations of sites implanted with intraoral autologous bone grafts or allografts. 15 human case reports. J Periodontol 1996;67:1025-33.

[37] Becker W, Becker BE, Caffesse R. A comparison of demin-eralized freeze-dried bone and autologous bone to induce bone formation in human extraction sockets. J Periodontol 1994;65:1128-33.

[38] Toeroek R, Dohan Ehrenfest DM The concept of Screw-Guided Bone Regeneration (S-GBR). Part 3: Fast ScrewGuided Bone Regeneration (FS-GBR) in the severely resorbed preimplant posterior mandible using allograft and Leukocyte- and Platelet-Rich Fibrin (L PRF): a 4-year follow-up. POSEIDO. 2013; 1(2): 93-100.

[39] Nacopoulos C, Dontas I, Lelovas P, Galanos A, Vesalas AM, Raptou P, Mastoris M, Chronopoulos E, Papaioannou N. Enhancement of bone regeneration with the combination of platelet-rich fibrin and synthetic graft. J Craniofac Surg 2014; 25: 2164-2168.

[40] Del Corso M, Dohan Ehrenfest DM. Immediate implantation and peri-implant Natural Bone Regeneration (NBR) in the severely resorbed posterior mandible using Leukocyte- and Platelet-Rich Fibrin (L-PRF): a 4-year follow-up. POSEIDO. 2013;1(2):109-16.

[41] Joseph V R, Sam G, Amol NV. Clinical evaluation of autologous platelet rich fibrin in horizontal alveolar bony defects. J Clin Diagn Res 2014; 8: ZC43-ZC47.

[42] Hehn J, Schwenk T, Striegel M, et al. The effect of PRF (platelet-rich fibrin) inserted with a split-flap technique on soft tissue thickening and initial marginal bone loss around implants: Results of a randomized, controlled clinical trial. International Journal of Implant Dentistry. 2016;2(1):13

[43] Hamzacebi B, Oduncuoglo B, Alaaddinogl EE. Treatment of peri-implant bone defects with platelet-rich fibrin. Int J Periodont Restorative Dent 2015; 35(3): 414-422.

[44] Boora P, Rathee M, Bhoria M. Effect of Platelet Rich Fibrin (PRF) on peri-implant soft tissue and crestal bone in one-stage implant placement: a randomized controlled trial. J Clin Diagn Res 2015;9(4):ZC18-21.

[45] Oncu E, Alaaddinoglu EE. The effect of platelet-rich fibrin on implant stability. Int J Oral Maxillofac Implants 2015;30(3):578-82.

[46] Oncu E, Erbeyoglu AA. Enhancement of immediate implant stability and recovery using platelet-rich fibrin. Int J Periodontics Restorative Dent 2017.

[47] Rao SG, Bhat P, Nagesh KS, Rao GHR, Mirle B, Kharbhari L, Gangaprasad B. Bone Regeneration in Extraction Sockets with Autologous Platelet Rich Fibrin Gel. J. Maxillofac. Oral Surg 2013, 12(1): 11-16

[48] Del Corso M, Mazor Z, Rutkowski JL, Dohan Ehrenfest DM. The use of leukocyte- and platelet-rich fibrin during immediate post extractive implantation and loading for the esthetic replacement of a fractured maxillary central incisor. J Oral Implantol 2012; 38: 181-187.

[49] Gül en U, Sentürk MF, Mehdiyev. Flap-free treatment of an oro-antral communication with platelet-rich fibrin. The British Association of Oral and Maxillofacial Surgeons. Accepted 30 September 2015.

[50] Agarwal B, Pandey S, Roychoudhury A. New technique for closure of an oroantral fistula using platelet-rich fibrin. Br J Oral Maxillofacial Surg 2016; 54: e31–e32.

[51] Borgonovo AE, Berardinelli FV, Favale M, et al. Surgical options in oroantral fistula treatment. The Open Dentistry Journal. 2012;6:94-98

[52] Del Fabbro M, Gallesio G, Mozzati M. Autologous platelet concentrates for bisphosphonate-related osteonecrosis of the jaw treatment and prevention. A systematic review of the literature. European Journal of Cancer. 2015;51(1):62-74

[53] Soydan SS, Uckan S. Management of bisphosphonaterelated osteonecrosis of the jaw with a platelet-rich fibrin membrane: technical report. J Oral Maxillofac Surg 2014; 72: 322-326.

[54] Shawky H, Seifeldin SA. Does platelet-rich fibrin enhance bone quality and quantity of alveolar cleft reconstruction? Cleft Palate Craniofac J 2016;53(5):597-606.

[55] Geeta IB, Galagali G, Kulkarni S, Suran P, Noushin F. A natural meliorate: Revolutionary tissue engineering in endodontics. J Clin Diagn Res. 2013; 7:2644-6.

[56] Shivashankar VY, Johns DA, Vidyanath S, Kumar MR. Platelet rich fibrin in the revitalization of tooth with necrotic pulp and open apex. J Conserv Dent. 2012;15:395-8.

[57] Jayalakshmi KB, Agarwal S, Singh MP, Vishwanath BT, Krishna A, Agrawal R et al. Platelet-rich fibrin with βtricalcium phosphate-A noval approach for bone augmentation in chronic periapical lesion: A Case report. Case Rep Dent. 2012; 2012:902858.

[58] Nagaveni NB, Poornima P, Joshi JS, Pathak S, Nandini DB. Revascularization of Immature, Nonvital Permanent Tooth Using Platelet-rich Fibrin in Children. Pediatr Dent 2015;37:E1-E6

[59] Sundar JS, Varma KM, Kalyan Satish RK, Sajjan GS, Tanikonda R. A Biological Approach in Repair of Damaged Dental Pulp and Periapical Tissues using Platelet Rich Fibrin, Mineral Trioxide Aggregate and Laser

Bio stimulation. IJSS Case Reports & Reviews 2015; 1(11): 44-50

[60] Kiran NK, Mukunda KS, Tilak Raj TN (2011) Platelet concentrates: A promising innovation in dentistry. J Dent Sci Res 2: 50-61.

[61] Kawase T, Kamiya M, Kobayashi M, Tanaka T, Okuda K, et al. (2015) The heat-compression technique for the conversion of platelet-rich fibrin preparation to a barrier mem Platelet-rich fibrin. Int J ClinExp Med 8: 7922-7929.

[62] Cortellini P, Tonetti MS, Lang NP, Lindhe J (2008) Regenerative periodontal therapy. Clinical Periodontology and Implant Dentistry (5th edn.). Forlaget Munksgaard, Copenhagen. pp: 902-954.

[63] Bansal C, Bharti V. Evaluation of efficacy of autologous platelet-rich fibrin with demineralized-freeze dried bone allograft in the treatment of periodontal intrabony defects. Journal of Indian Society of Periodontology. 2013;17:361-366. DOI: 10.4103/0972-124X.115663

[64] Goldman MJ, Ross IF, Goteiner D. Effect of periodontal therapy on patients maintained for 15 years or longer. A retrospective study. Journal of Periodontology. 1986;57:347-353. DOI: 10.1902/jop.1986.57.6.347

[65] Desarda HM, Gurav AN, Gaikwad SP, Inamdar SP. Platelet rich fibrin: a new hope for regeneration in aggressive periodontitis patients: report of two cases. Indian J Dent Res 2013; 24: 627-630.

[66] Jankovic S, Aleksic Z, Klokkevold P, Lekovic V, Dimitrijevic B, et al. (2012) Use of platelet-rich fibrin membrane following treatment of gingival recession: a randomized clinical trial. Int J Periodontics Restorative Dent 32: 41-50.

[67] Kumar G, Murthy K (2013) A comparative evaluation of sub epithelial connective tissue graft (SCTG) versus platelet concentrate graft (PCG) in the treatment of gingival recession using coronally advanced flap technique: a 12-month study. J Indian Soc Periodontol 17: 771-776.

[68] Aravindaksha SP, Batra P, Sood V, Kumar A, Gupta GT. Use of Platelet-Rich Fibrin Membrane as a Palatal Bandage. Clin Adv Periodontics 2014; 4:246-250.

[69] Femminella B, Iaconi MC, Di Tullio M, Romano L, Sinjari B, D'Arcangelo C, De Ninis P, Paolantonio M. Clinical Comparison of Platelet-Rich Fibrin and a Gelatin Sponge in the Management of Palatal Wounds After Epithelialized Free Gingival Graft Harvest: A Randomized Clinical Trial. J Periodontol 2016;87:103-113.

Chapter 5

Emerging Role of Nuclear Medicine in Oral and Maxillofacial Surgery

Tina Nazerani, Peter Kalmar and Reingard M. Aigner

Abstract

During the past several years, nuclear medicine has emerged as one of the most useful imaging studies in oral and maxillofacial surgery, not only in diagnosis and staging but also in the management plan and follow-up protocols of many cancer or inflammatory diseases. Nuclear medicine has in addition a special place in treating several benign and malignant diseases. The practicing maxillofacial surgeon's knowledge of nuclear medicine capabilities and advantages and disadvantages of each modality is crucial in his or her daily work. The purpose of this chapter is to clarify the important role of nuclear medicine in diagnosis and treatment of oral and maxillofacial region pathologies as well as its indications and limitations in the daily practice of the oral and maxillofacial surgeon.

Keywords: nuclear medicine, maxillofacial surgery, oral cancer, bone scintigraphy, SPECT/CT, sentinel lymph node, F18-FDG, PET/CT

1. Introduction

Nuclear medicine has become one of the essential diagnostic tools in all fields of medicine, and one of these fields is oral and maxillofacial surgery. As an independent specialty, it is characterized by the injection of radioactive labeled materials to identify the presence and location of primary and metastatic cancer, inflammatory diseases, etc. Advanced imaging procedures such as positron emission tomography (PET) combined with computed tomography (CT) as well as single-photon emission computerized tomography (SPECT) and sentinel lymph node scintigraphy have shown to be precise diagnostic tools in oral/maxillofacial pathologies; however its importance and role in diagnosis of pathological conditions need to be discussed more and better presented to other medical and surgical disciplines [1].

In comparison to other morphological imaging modalities such as CT, magnetic resonance imaging (MRI), and ultrasonography, biochemical changes in different tissues of various pathophysiological processes are diagnosed earlier by radionuclide imaging through the injection of radioactively labeled substances [2].

2. A short journey throughout history

Chemistry Nobel Prize winner Georg Charles de Hevesy was the first to use radioactive isotopes to study the metabolic processes of plants and animals.

He observed the chemical activity of the animal body by replacing parts of stable isotopes with small amounts of radioactive isotopes. In 1923, he published his first study of radioactive tracer Lead-212 to observe the uptake of labeled ions by the different parts of horse bean. He carried out his experiments in animals with Bismuth-210, injecting it intramuscularly in rabbits to follow the dynamic behavior of the tracer. De Hevesy is often referred to as the father of nuclear medicine [3].

However, one must not forget that the history of nuclear medicine is full of contributions by other scientists such as Wilhelm Konrad Roentgen, Marie Curie, and Henri Becquerel.

Hermann Blumgart was the first to perform human use of radioactive tracers in 1925. He measured the "velocity of the circulation" by measuring the time it took the injected solutions of radon flow from one arm to another. George Moore, MD, a neurosurgeon at the University of Minnesota, performed the first brain study using Di-iodofluorescein to detect brain tumors [4].

Nuclear medicine's golden era of recognition by the medical community began in 1946, when it was described as a successful treatment of thyroid cancer using radioiodine (I-131). This is considered to be one of the turning points in the history of nuclear medicine [5].

The modern principle of nuclear medicine is based on the works of Benedict Cassena and Hal O. Anger for developing the first rectilinear scanner and scintillation camera. Three-dimensional reconstruction of the heart in the 1980s using SPECT has led to the establishment of nuclear medicine in cardiology by using radiotracers for the diagnosis of various heart diseases.

The most recent development is the invention of PET/CT. This modality plays a pivotal role in all stages of oncological diseases from pre-treatment staging to the follow-up protocols [6].

3. Statistics, etiology, and pathology of head and neck cancers

The core principle of every living creature is in the so-called condition of homeostasis, which allows biomolecules to balance themselves in a dynamic process. When homeostasis is disrupted, it can lead to an unbalanced situation or, in other words, disease. The tracers with similar chemical structures as the ones present in the body are used to understand and analyze the in vivo molecular situation of one organ or several organs.

The growing need for a precise diagnostic workup has led to a search for more center-based instead of disease-based patients.

Modern medicine today prescribes a complete survey of the disease process, locating cancer and possible metastatic growths, before taking an action, i.e., surgery or chemo-radioactive ablations.

According to the 2018 global cancer statistics, lip and oral cavity cancers are the leading areas of tumor involvement in the head and neck region. They are followed by nasopharynx, oropharynx, hypopharynx, and salivary glands. These types of cancer are more prevalent in men. Global incidence rate is higher in Southern Asia, especially in Sri Lanka and India, where it is the leading cause of death in male patients [7]. The risk factors for head and neck cancers are tobacco and alcohol [8–11]. The risk is even higher in cases using both alcohol and tobacco than cases using either alcohol or tobacco alone [12–14].

Squamous cell carcinoma (SCC) is the most common type of cancer in the head and neck region, with a rate of over 90%, and mostly found in the larynx and oral cavity. The other cancer types are salivary glands adenocarcinomas, melanoma, lymphomas, and rare tumors (e.g., paragangliomas) [15].

Nearly one third of patients are seen in early stages, while the remaining two thirds present in advanced stages.

Surgery and/or radiotherapy seems to be more useful in early stages; however, due to the high risk of recurrence and metastasis as well as the development of second primary cancer, the prognosis of these cases is also not significantly better [16].

Carcinogenic subtypes of human papillomavirus (HPV), especially subtype 16, are associated with some head and neck cancers commonly involving oropharynx, tonsil, and the base of the tongue [17–19].

Poor oral hygiene, preserved and/or salted foods, and occupational exposure to certain industrial materials such as asbestos are other risk factors in nasopharyngeal and laryngeal cancers. In addition, radiation exposure is a risk factor in salivary gland cancers. Epstein-Barr virus is responsible for cancer of the nasopharynx and salivary glands [20–23].

4. Imaging studies in nuclear medicine

The desire to find the best therapeutic management and oncologic regimens is undeniable. To exactly determine the stage of the cancer in head and neck area is indispensable to the oncological team for choosing the best treatment strategy as well as follow-up protocols.

Radionuclide imaging studies are as follows:

a. Bone scintigraphy

b. Statistics and indications

c. PET/CT scans

d. Lymphoscintigraphy

5. Bone scintigraphy in head and neck surgery

The bone is in a constant state of turnover as a result of metabolic or mechanical demands, and a fine balance is present between osteogenesis and bone resorption. Oral pathologies cause metabolic changes in the bone and surrounding structures of maxillofacial region; these changes can be due to trauma, infection, neoplasm, or other etiologies. These disease processes are associated with hypervascularization and biochemical changes of the bone and surrounding structures; therefore, it is of great value to use bone scintigraphy with its minimal radiation exposure to identify these disease processes.

The conventional X-ray is still the most convenient method for detection of pathologies affecting boney structure of the maxillofacial region. However, the changes are first seen when more than 30% of bone structure is involved.

On the other hand, morphological changes due to the biochemical processes of osteoblastic activities can be detected at the early stages of bone remodeling by bone scintigraphy [1].

Bone scintigraphy is a functional imaging study, whereas other anatomical modalities, such as CT or MRI, are structural studies.

Bone scintigraphy can detect osteoblastic activity with only a 10% change above the normal value. Although the quality and resolution of bone scans are not as sharp as X-ray, abnormalities can be seen long before morphological changes. Bone scintigraphy is also helpful in cases with suspected non-vitality bone lesions.

Most of the pathological processes involving the bone are the result of new bone formation or increased turnover. These appear in bone scans as areas of increased tracer uptake, known as "hot spots."

Inactive metabolic conditions decreased or lack of new bone formation or reduced blood supply result in decreased tracer uptake showing either a disruptive reparative process or suggesting an aggressive lesion of nonconformity to the native tissues. "Cold spots" are areas with a lack of or reduced tracer uptake.

Bone scintigraphy is done by intravenous injection of Technetium-99m-labeled diphosphonate with 140 KeV gamma energy. It has a short physical half-life of 6 h with minimal radiation exposure.

A significant amount of unbound tracer is excreted in the urine. The tracer has a high ratio of up to 40% affinity to the hydroxyapatite.

Depending on the clinical diagnosis, there are different techniques for performing a bone scan. The "planar whole-body" images are the anterior and posterior acquisition of the skeleton. This includes static images 3–4 h after tracer injection. If necessary, an additional "spot view" can be obtained.

"Three-phase" bone scintigraphy consists of the blood flow and the soft tissue images and "delayed static images." Dynamic images are acquired during the intravenous injection of the tracer and demonstrate the vascular phase by assessment of the tracer inflow. The next phase, 5–10 min after injection, known as blood pool phase, consists of image acquisition of tracer distribution of the soft tissues in the region of interest. It reflects tissue distribution of the tracer, especially hyperemia. The next phase consists of delayed images, 3–4 h after injection, when the maximal uptake of the tracer is present. The "whole-body" or "focal static" images are acquired at this time. The three-phase bone scan is indicated in primary bone tumors, trauma, or infectious/inflammatory processes.

Bone scintigraphy is indicated for diagnosis and follow-up of several conditions such as malignancy, infection and inflammatory processes, temporomandibular joint disorder, cystic change, activity of mandibular condyle hyperplasia, and viability of bone grafts.

5.1 Statistics and indications in maxillofacial surgery

Maxilla and mandible are common sites that are affected by neoplasms such as sarcomas and carcinomas. Sarcomas are originated from the mesenchymal part of the jaw. In contrast, the carcinomas can originate either by the locoregional lesions of the oral mucosa or as metastasis of a primary tumor such as adenocarcinomas of the breast, prostate, thyroid, colon, and uterus.

Metastases are the cause of up to 8% of oral malignancies. Due to bone marrow scarcity in the maxilla and mandible, less than 1% of oral malignancies are bone metastases.

In the oral region, etiologies such as osteomyelitis, trauma, and osteoarthritis can also lead to positive bone scans. Chronic osteomyelitis is a challenge especially in the differential diagnosis of the oral and maxillofacial primary cancers [24] (**Figure 1**).

5.2 Bone scintigraphy in osteomyelitis

There are different types of osteomyelitis of the jaw which can be divided into purulent, osteoradionecrosis, and noninfectious (diffuse sclerosing osteomyelitis).

DOI: http://dx.doi.org/10.5772/intechopen.92278

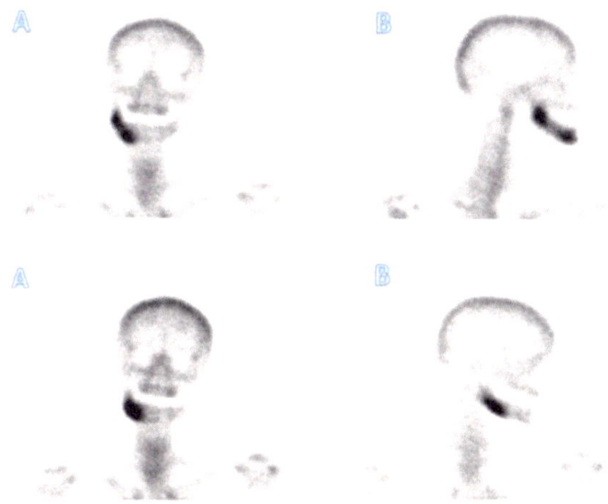

Figure 1.
Bone scintigraphy of a patient with chronic osteomyelitis shows elevated osteoblastic activity as a result of infection in the angle of mandible and mental protuberance of the right jawbone. The lower row of pictures shows the reduction of the involved area after antibiotic therapy and multiple bone curettages. (A) Anterior view and (B) lateral view.

Medication-related osteonecrosis (MRONJ) of the jaw is another subtype of osteomyelitis which is on the rise [25].

MRONJ is a difficult clinical diagnosis in the field of maxillofacial surgery and dentistry. It results from drugs that have anti-bone resorption effects such as denosumab or antiangiogenic medications like sorafenib and also in patients undergoing bisphosphonate therapy. This complication occurs only in the jaw bones. According to some studies, the incidence of MRONJ is around 12%. Due to the rising number of bisphosphonate therapy, over a million prescriptions a year in USA, the exact knowledge of this complication, is essential.

The typical clinical features are painful jaw swelling, loosening of teeth, or extrusion of the jawbone [26–28].

At the early stage of the disease, conservative approach such as pain killers and antibiotics is the treatment of choice, whereas in advanced stages, due to bone exposure, infection, necrosis, and other bone-related complications, surgical intervention such as debridement or resection should be considered [27].

Bone scintigraphy has proved to be a useful diagnostic tool in the early stages of MRONJ. It has the sensitivity of 67% and specificity of 79% in early asymptomatic stages in patients with castration-resistant prostate carcinoma under bisphosphonate therapy [29].

Although several studies show the high detection rate of MRONJ in bone scans, it is still not the routine diagnostic modality in daily practice [30, 31]. However, it should be considered not only for staging or follow-up but also to control the bone status of the jaw (**Figure 2**).

5.3 Bone scintigraphy in fibrous dysplasia

Fibrous dysplasia (FD) is a rare benign lesion in young patients. Fibro-osseous tissue replaces the healthy tissues causing bone overgrowth; sometimes it regresses after adulthood. It could be monostotic (single bone involvement) or polyostotic (more than one bone involvement). Craniofacial bones are mostly prone to be involved. It can be asymptomatic or presents itself with bone malformation,

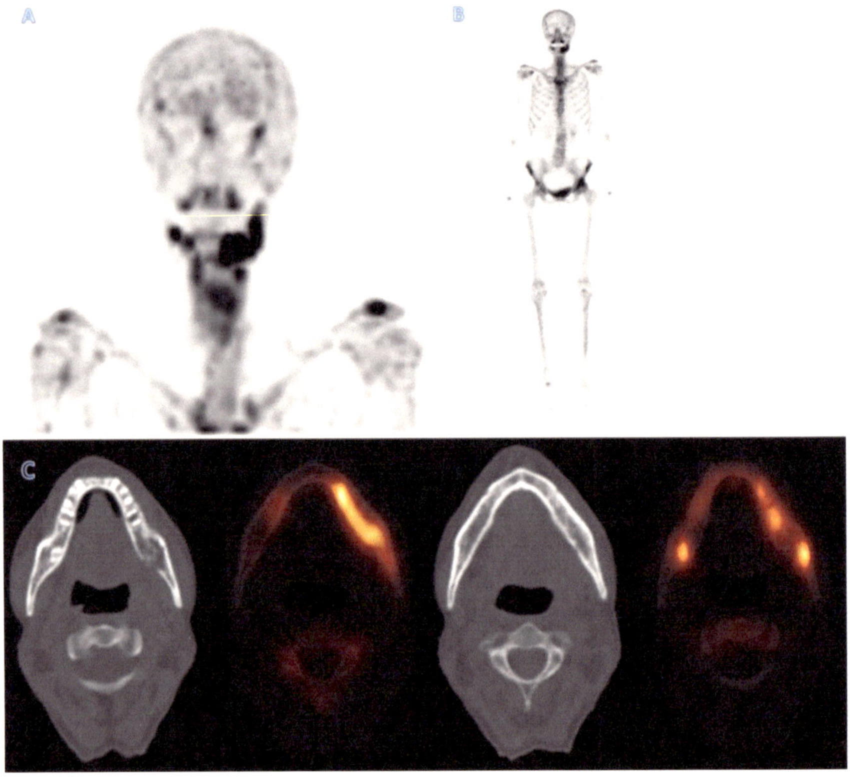

Figure 2.
(A) Bone scintigraphy in a patient after tonsillectomy due to squamous cell carcinoma and chemo radiotherapy with osteonecrosis of the mandible. The osteoblastic activity is visualized in both sides of the mandible. The hot spots show osteoblastic activity in the jaw. (B) Whole-body scan confirms negative bone metastases in the skeleton. (C) SPECT/CT images show the combination of anatomical and biological images.

pain, or pathological fractures. Several studies show the significant technetium 99m-methylene/diethylene diphosphonate (MDP/DPD) uptake on the bone scan.

FD requires long-term medical observation. Surgery is needed when there are signs of bone deformation, pain, compression of the nerve, or malignancy transformation. The probability of malignancy is less than 1%, and it occurs primarily in patients with the history of radiotherapy (**Figure 3**).

Fibrous dysplasia imitates malignancy, especially in patients with previous history of cancer, and can be a difficult differential diagnosis; the exact diagnosis and knowledge of its radiological features can prevent unnecessary workup and possible unnecessary intervention [32].

5.4 Bone scintigraphy and Paget

Single-photon emission tomography/computed tomography (SPECT/CT) is another radionuclide imaging study and is used to visualize three-dimensional multiplanar tracer distribution in the region of interest with CT using an integrated CT scanner [33].

With the aid of SPECT/CT, the exact anatomical location and pathological metabolism can be assessed.

Paget's disease of the bone is a pathological metabolic condition, with abnormal bone resorption. An intense osteoblastic activity is the hallmark of the disease. Some patients are asymptomatic, whereas others present with bone deformity, pain, pathological fractures, osteoarthritis, and rarely neoplasm. Due to high

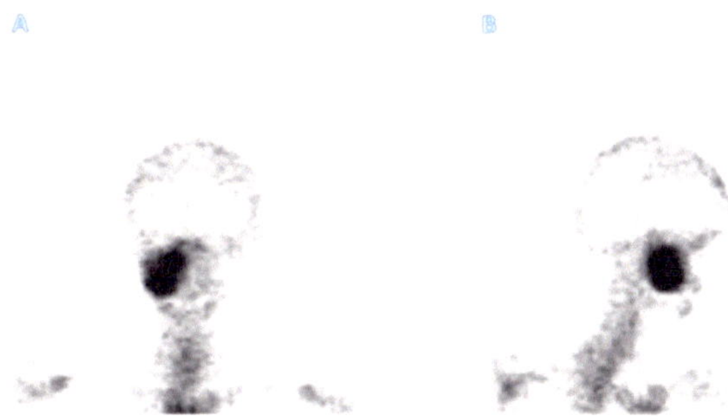

Figure 3.
Bone scintigraphy in a patient with fibrous dysplasia of the right maxilla. It shows the significant high radionuclide uptake, which also may be seen in bone malignancies with high osteoblastic activity. (A) Anterior view and (B) lateral view.

Bone scintigraphy	
Indications	• Specific bone diseases ○ Oncology (e.g., bone tumors and bone dysplasia) ○ Rheumatology (e.g., osteonecrosis of the jaw) ○ Bone and join infection (acute, subacute or chronic osteomyelitis, malignant external otitis) ○ Traumatology and orthopedics ○ Metabolic bone disorders (skeletal manifestation of rare endocrine disorder such as acromegaly and hyperthyroidism) • To investigate unclear symptoms ○ Subacute or chronic musculoskeletal or bone pain with normal clinical examination and radiographs i. Arthralgia, bone pain localized or multifocal ○ As a complementary diagnostic tool in cases of abnormal biological and radiological abnormalities ○ Exclusion of osteomyelitis in case of fever of unknown origin • Metabolic assessment prior to therapy ○ Evaluation of osteoblastic activity before initiating treatment with bisphosphonates
Absolute and relative contraindications	• There is no absolute contraindication. In general, in nuclear medicine, scans are not suitable for pregnant women; the benefit versus risk should be considered and discussed • Breastfeeding should be interrupted for 4 h
Disadvantages	• Low specificity in bone disorders • Limitation of the technique in certain diseases • Not easily accessible
Advantages	• Higher sensitivity in bone disorders • Early detection of bone physiology and pathology

Table 1.
Brief overview of indications, contraindications, advantages, and disadvantages of bone scintigraphy.

osteoblastic activity, significant tracer uptake is visualized on bone scan. In the case of mandibular involvement, it may cause a total involvement of the mandible. In this case, it is called "black beard," which demonstrates the tracer uptake in the entire jawbone.

Unilateral condylar hyperplasia (UCH) is a rare pathological growth of the mandibular condyle, during growth phase in adolescence. Facial asymmetry, malocclusion, deformity, and sometimes pain and temporomandibular joint dysfunction are the common clinical features. Condylar hyperplasia is a self-limiting status; however, due to the unproportioned growth of one condylar, it always results in one-sided facial asymmetry. The growth phase is classified into two phases: active phase and stationary phase. The mandibular asymmetry is highly correlated to the active phase. Routine imaging modalities such as X-rays and CT show anatomical changes. Bone scintigraphy alone or in combination with SPECT can provide both anatomical and functional information, especially in the early stages of the disease before any morphological changes are visible.

Morphological imaging modalities should be used in combination with bone scintigraphy, which provides information on osteoblastic activity. For example, in case of condylar hyperplasia, bone scintigraphy can determine if the growth has stopped before any treatment implemented. Symmetrical uptake in both sides of the jawbone shows no more progression, and therefore treatment can be undertaken.

Early detection of bone physiology and pathology is the greatest advantage of bone scintigraphy, which makes it more sensitive than X-rays. However, its low specificity is its disadvantage. Combining the interpretation of both procedures may decrease their limitations (**Table 1**).

The extension of benign bone lesions such as odontogenic myxoma, keratocyst, and ameloblastoma can be determined by bone scintigraphy. The radionuclide tracer uptake is usually elevated, and the bony changes may be significantly more prominent, compared to X-ray. This information helps the treatment by planning a more extended resection and therefore prevents recurrence.

Bone scintigraphy has its own advantages and disadvantages. It is the responsibility of maxillofacial team to orchestrate imaging modalities in order to decide on the best treatment and to plan follow-up [32].

6. PET/CT scan and oromaxillofacial tumors

As an advanced screening method, PET/CT can detect exact anatomical extension as well as the biological behavior of the tumor.

The fundamental characteristic of human malignancies is the overexpression of the glucose transporter, especially in HNSCC (**Figure 4**).

It can be assessed by high glucose metabolism in the tumors with F18-2-fluoro-2 deoxy-D-glucose (FDG) and PET/CT known as FDG-PET/CT (**Figure 5**).

The combination of PET and CT enables immediate sequential detection of metabolic (FDG-PET) and morphological (CT) information by one examination. Although various methods for retrospective co-registration of PET and CT images have been available since the 1980s, PET/CT imaging has only recently been clinically established through the availability of combined PET/CT (**Table 2**).

In summary PET/CT scan indications are as follows:

a. Differentiating benign from malignant lesions.

b. Search for an unknown primary tumor if metastasis is the first tumor manifestation or if paraneoplastic syndrome is present.

c. Staging of a known tumor condition.

d. Determine response to therapy in the case of known tumors.

e. Assessing the presence of residual tumor disease (vital tumor tissue vs. scar tissue).

f. Determining recurrence, for example, with increasing tumor marker concentration.

g. Selecting exact site for biopsy.

h. Help with radiotherapy planning and non-oncological issues (e.g., infection) [34].

However, it is not yet a gold standard technique according to most guidelines.

Head and neck cancers (HNC) are responsible for approximately 4% of all cancers in the United States. The survival rate in the early stages is up to 80%, whereas in advanced stages, the survival rate can be lower than 40% [35, 36].

Initial assessments of local tumor extension and regional lymph node involvement are of critical importance in head and neck squamous cell carcinoma (HNSCC) and in implementing the most appropriate treatment.

Physical examination, fiber optic endoscopy, CT, and MRI are initial steps to access the local extension of the primary tumor and the regional lymph node status [37]. Recently, positron emission tomography/computed tomography (PET/CT) has found its place in the early workup diagnosis in HNSCC due to its whole-body imaging capability.

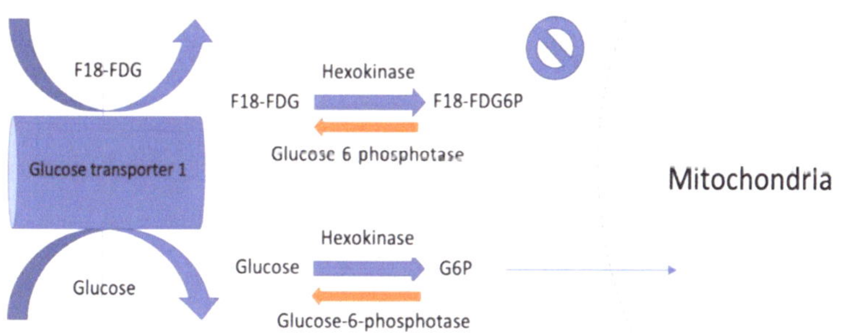

Figure 4.
Schematic of the metabolic trapping of F18-FDG in a tumor cell showing the trapping mechanism in FDG imaging. The glucose transporter 1 (GLUT1) serves as a channel for its uptake. It accumulates in tumor cells, where the metabolism by hexokinase and glucose-6-phosphatase takes place. FDG will be phosphorylated by hexokinase. Glucose-6-phosphotase (G6Pase) counteracts hexokinase phosphorylation by converting glucose-6-phosphate (G6P) to glucose. Therefore, high G6Pase activity leads the accelerated conversion of FDG-6-phosphate (FDG6P) to its FDG form, as a result, the uptake reduces, and it will be released from the cell.

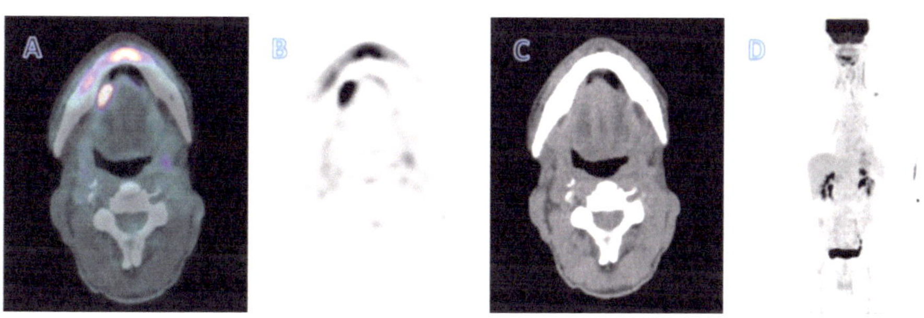

Figure 5.
PET/CT with F18-FDG shows the high metabolism in the lesion in the floor of the mouth, without any local and remote metastasis in stem-body scan. (A) Fusion image, (B) PET, (C) CT, and (D) stem-body scan.

According to different studies, the PET/CT can change the course of pre-treatment, TNM classification, as well as therapeutic management by 31–43% in comparison to conventional workup diagnoses especially in patients with advanced stages of HNSCC (stages III and IV) [37–39] (**Figure 6**).

Thus, its clinical impact is not limited to malignancies of the maxillofacial region. The clinical role of FDG-PET/CT in dental implantology has shown its usefulness in implant monitoring, especially in understanding the implant loss. The most common cause of implant loss is peri-implantitis possibly due to infectious and inflammatory etiologies. Benouaich et al. discussed the relevance of FDG-PET/CT diagnosis in implantology. In their study, they showed that the

PET/CT	
Indications	• Primary diagnostic: unknown primary malignancy, differentiation • Staging pre-treatment and on presentation: nasopharyngeal cancer • Evaluation of the treatment response: • Restaging in case of relapse • Radiotherapy planning of malignant and benign lesions
Absolute and relative contraindications	• There is no absolute contraindication. In general, in nuclear medicine, scans are not suitable for pregnant women; the benefit versus risk should be considered and discussed • Breastfeeding should be interrupted for 4 h
Disadvantages	• No specificity for tumor types • Chances of false positive especially in infection-inflammation • Very small lesion under 5 mm can be missed • Radiation exposure
Advantages	• Several tumors • It provides whole-body imaging, which allows for the exploration of distant metastasis • It has a high resolution • High accuracy because of combined CT images • High sensitivity depending on metabolic activity • Well tolerated

Table 2.
A brief overview of indications, contraindications, advantages, and disadvantages of PET/CT.

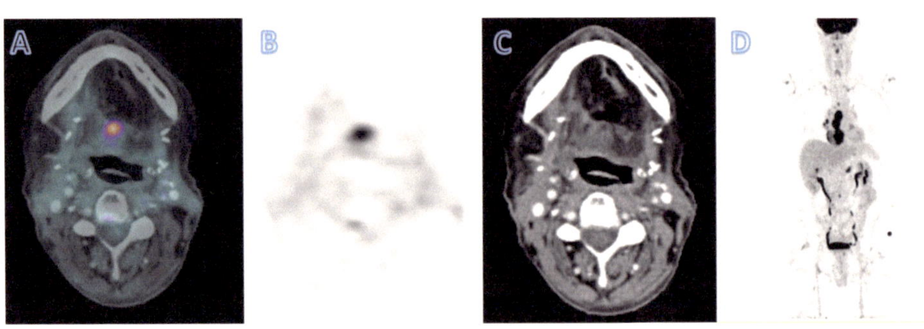

Figure 6.
PET/CT with F18-FDG shows the pathological activity in the residual tongue after partial resection. The stem-body scan demonstrates the hypermetabolic active mediastinal and thoracic lymph nodes as well as a single lumbar bone metastasis. (A) Fusion image, (B) PET, (C) CT, and (D) stem-body scan.

FDG-PET/CT plays an essential role in differentiating normal osseointegration of an implant from peri-implantitis. As a result of the pathological hypermetabolism of the peri-implant, it can be identified by FDG-PET/CT, leading to corresponding treatment [40].

7. Lymphoscintigraphy and sentinel lymph node in oral and maxillofacial surgery

Sentinel lymph node was first described in 1980s when Donald L. Morton, a surgeon at the John Wayne Cancer Center in Santa Monika, and his pathologist Alistair J. Cochran suggested the idea of lymph node mapping with biopsy of the sentinel lymph node in melanoma. They described the sentinel lymph node as the first node, which is the first portal in the diseased cell migration from the lesion. They proposed the importance of the first node on the localization of the lesion. In their paper they emphasized that a "sentinel node" is the initial lymph node upon which the primary tumor drains. Today we know that the sentinel lymph node is the first node on the lymphatic pathway that drains directly from the tumor [41].

SLNB was initially used in melanoma and breast cancer. The indications are melanoma with Breslow thickness up to 1mm, high-risk squamous cell carcinoma, and Merkel carcinoma. Due to the anatomical complexity of the lymphatic pathways in the head and neck region, its importance has been recently appreciated in oncology. To avoid unnecessary neck dissection to decrease the morbidity and improve the patient's quality of life, it is suggested to perform SLNB also in head and neck cancer patients.

Cervical lymph node involvement status is the crucial deciding element in staging, management and predicting prognosis in patients with head and neck SCC.

Recent studies have shown the potential of SLNB as a minimally invasive procedure for assessing occult metastasis and thus reducing morbidity in patients undergoing elective neck dissection (END). Its reliability in T1-T2N0 in the oral cavity and oropharyngeal cancers has been validated for more than a decade, yet till today there is no consensus reached as to when and on whom to perform.

In the field of nuclear medicine, the sentinel lymph node is the first node that is visible after the administration of the tracer. Flow imaging or "dynamic phase" is the first phase, immediately after injection, which shows the lymphatic pathway and clearance. In the late stage also known as the "static phase", can the very first node or sometimes more than one node be visualized and anatomically pinpointed.

Lymphatic mapping is performed with either radiolabeled tracers or vital blue dye (VBD). In conventional lymphoscintigraphy, the main tracer is technetium 99m-labeled radio colloids. The most widely used radiotracer in the United States is technetium 99m-sulfur colloid, and in Europe technetium 99m-albumin-based-nano colloid is used. They both, however, lack optimal rapid clearance of the injection site, high accumulation within the first node, and minimal tracer uptake in the distant nodes [42].

Recently, to overcome the limitations of the conventional colloid tracers, a new tracer has been developed to fulfill the aforementioned shortcomings. Technetium 99m-diethylenetriaminepentaacetic acid (DTPA)-mannosyl-dextran (also known as 99mTc-tilmanocept) is a novel radiopharmaceutical agent that selectively binds to CD206 receptors, which presents in high concentration in lymph nodes on the membrane of macrophages and dendritic cells. Tilmanocept structure consists of a dextran main domain and the DTPA as well as mannose units which are attached to the central part. The average diameter of this macromolecule is 7nm. The mannose binds to the CD206 receptor, whereas the DTPA serves as the binding part for

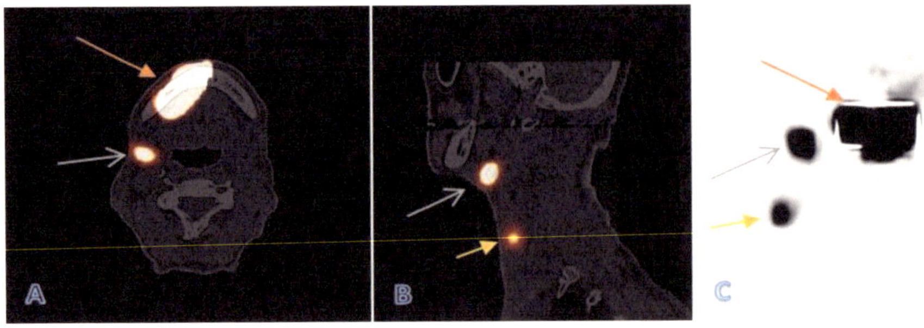

Figure 7.
Sentinel node scintigraphy in a patient with SCC of the soft tissue between the body of mandible and the hyoid bone (orange arrow) and negative clinical examination as well as normal lymph node status in MRI. To avoid radical neck dissection sentinel node scintigraphy has been performed to detect the nodes with direct drainage from the lesion. After 60 min, two cervical lymph nodes were visualized (white and yellow arrows). (A) Axial view, (B) sagittal view, and (C) planar image.

technetium 99m. Due to its small size, it has a rapid uptake in lymph nodes, and its targeted binding prevents its migration to distal nodes [43, 44].

Recent studies have shown the high sensitivity and specificity of up to 94% of tilmanocept in patients with head and neck squamous cell carcinoma [45, 46]. Assessment of single-photon emission computed tomography with computed tomography (SPECT/CT) in addition to planar lymph scintigraphy provides precise anatomical localization in clinically negative nodal status and early stages of the head and neck cancers [24] (**Figure 7**).

8. Conclusion

Diagnosis of cancer and inflammatory diseases and the differentiation between the two are of utmost importance. Nuclear medicine by using radionuclide substances can detect the dynamic aspect of a disease process, and when this dynamic study is mingled by a morphological study, CT or MRI, the management team can see a clearer picture of the disease process and plan treatment protocols accordingly. Sentinel lymph node biopsy is gaining momentum in cancer treatment protocols as a MUST-DO procedure before the definitive treatment plan is implemented.

Conflict of interest

The authors declare no conflict of interest.

Author details

Tina Nazerani*, Peter Kalmar and Reingard M. Aigner
Division of Nuclear Medicine, Department of Radiology, Medical University of Graz, Graz, Austria

*Address all correspondence to: tina.nazerani-hooshmand@medunigraz.at

References

[1] Baur DA et al. Nuclear medicine in oral and maxillofacial diagnosis: A review for the practicing dental professional. The Journal of Contemporary Dental Practice. 2004;**5**(1):94-104. DOI: 10.5005/jcdp-5-1-94

[2] Shreenivasamurthy P, Shastry SL. Nuclear medicine in orofacial diagnosis: A review. Journal of Medicine, Radiology, Pathology and Surgery. 2016;**3**(4):12-16. DOI: 10.15713/ins.jmrps.63

[3] Medal GVH, Hevesy GV. Prize for nuclear medicine. International Journal of Nuclear Medicine and Biology. 1978;**5**(2-3):156. DOI: 10.1016/0047-0740(78)90053-0

[4] Wagner HN. Nuclear medicine: 100 years in the making. Journal of Nuclear Medicine. 1996;**37**(10):18N-37N

[5] Henkin RE et al. Nuclear medicine. Journal of Nuclear Medicine. 2007;**48**(5):846-846. DOI: 10.2967/jnumed.107.040329

[6] Society of Nuclear Medicine. The Benefits of Nuclear Medicine. 1995. Available from: http://interactive.snm.org/docs/whatisnucmed.pdf

[7] Bray F et al. Global Cancer Statistics 2018: GLOBOCAN estimates of incidence and mortality worldwide for 36 cancers in 185 Countries. CA: A Cancer Journal for Clinicians. 2018;**68**(6):394-424. DOI: 10.3322/caac.21492

[8] Gandini S et al. Tobacco smoking and cancer: A meta-analysis. International Journal of Cancer. 2007;**122**(1):155-164. DOI: 10.1002/ijc.23033

[9] Hashibe M. Evidence for an important role of alcohol- and aldehyde-metabolizing genes in cancers of the upper aerodigestive tract. Cancer Epidemiology Biomarkers & Prevention. 2006;**15**(4):696-703. DOI: 10.1158/1055-9965.epi-05-0710

[10] Hashibe M et al. Alcohol drinking in never users of tobacco, cigarette smoking in never drinkers, and the risk of head and neck cancer: Pooled analysis in the international head and neck cancer epidemiology consortium. JNCI Journal of the National Cancer Institute. 2007;**99**(10):777-789. DOI: 10.1093/jnci/djk179

[11] Boffetta P et al. Smokeless tobacco and cancer. The Lancet Oncology. 2008;**9**(7):667-675. DOI: 10.1016/s1470-2045(08)70173-6

[12] Mclaughlin JK et al. Dietary factors in oral and pharyngeal cancer. JNCI Journal of the National Cancer Institute. 1988;**80**(15):1237-1243. DOI: 10.1093/jnci/80.15.1237

[13] Tuyns A-J et al. Cancer of the larynx/hypopharynx, tobacco and alcohol: Iarc International Case-Control Study in Turin and Varese (Italy), Zaragoza and Navarra (Spain), Geneva (Switzerland) and Calvados (France). International Journal of Cancer. 1988;**41**(4):483-491. DOI: 10.1002/ijc.2910410403

[14] Hashibe M. Risk factors: Tobacco and alcohol. Epidemiology, Pathogenesis, and Prevention of Head and Neck Cancer. 2010:65-85. DOI: 10.1007/978-1-4419-1472-9_4

[15] Shah JP, Lydiatt W. Treatment of cancer of the head and neck. CA: A Cancer Journal for Clinicians. 1995;**45**(6):352-368. DOI: 10.3322/canjclin.45.6.352

[16] Heroiu Cataloiu AD, Danciu CE, Popescu CR. Multiple cancers of the head and neck. Maedica (Buchar). 2013;**8**(1):80-85

[17] Chaturvedi AK et al. Human papillomavirus and rising oropharyngeal cancer incidence in the United States. Journal of Clinical Oncology. 2011;**29**(32):4294-4301. DOI: 10.1200/jco.2011.36.4596

[18] Adelstein DJ et al. Head and neck squamous cell cancer and the human papillomavirus: Summary of a National Cancer Institute State of the Science Meeting, November 9-10, 2008, Washington, D.C. Head & Neck. 2009;**31**(11):1393-1422. DOI: 10.1002/hed.21269

[19] Gillison ML et al. Distinct risk factor profiles for human papillomavirus type 16–positive and human papillomavirus type 16–negative head and neck cancers. JNCI: Journal of the National Cancer Institute. 2008;**100**(6):407-420. DOI: 10.1093/jnci/djn025

[20] Yu MC, Yuan JM. Nasopharyngeal Cancer. In: Schottenfeld D, Fraumeni JF Jr, editors. Cancer Epidemiology and Prevention. 3rd ed. New York: Oxford University Press; 2006

[21] Yu MC, Yuan JM. Epidemiology of nasopharyngeal carcinoma. Seminars in Cancer Biology. 2002;**12**(6):421-429

[22] Hamilton-Dutoit SJ et al. Undifferentiated carcinoma of the salivary gland in greenlandic eskimos: Demonstration of Epstein-Barr virus DNA by in situ nucleic acid hybridization. Human Pathology. 1991;**22**(8):811-815. DOI: 10.1016/0046-8177(91)90210-g

[23] Leung SY et al. Lymphoepithelial carcinoma of the salivary gland: In situ detection of Epstein-Barr virus. Journal of Clinical Pathology. 1995;**48**(11):1022-1027. DOI: 10.1136/jcp.48.11.1022

[24] Toom IJD et al. The added value of SPECT-CT for the identification of sentinel lymph nodes in early stage oral cancer. European Journal of Nuclear Medicine and Molecular Imaging. 2017;**44**(6):998-1004. DOI: 10.1007/s00259-017-3613-8

[25] Kitagawa Y et al. Imaging modalities for drug-related osteonecrosis of the jaw (3), positron emission tomography imaging for the diagnosis of medication-related osteonecrosis of the jaw. Japanese Dental Science Review. 2019;**55**(1):65-70. DOI: 10.1016/j.jdsr.2018.12.001

[26] Arrain Y, Masud T. A current update on osteonecrosis of the jaw and bisphosphonates. Dental Update. 2011;**38**(10):672-678. DOI: 10.12968/denu.2011.38.10.672

[27] Ruggiero SL et al. American association of oral and maxillofacial surgeons position paper on medication-related osteonecrosis of the jaw—2014 update. Journal of Oral and Maxillofacial Surgery. 2014;**72**(10):1938-1956. DOI: 10.1016/j.joms.2014.04.031

[28] Scully's Medical Problems in Dentistry. 7th ed. London, United Kingdom: Churchill Livingstone; 2015

[29] Thomas C et al. Advantages and disadvantages of bone protective agents in metastatic prostate cancer: Lessons learned. Dentistry Journal. 2016;**4**(3):28. DOI: 10.3390/dj4030028

[30] O'ryan FS et al. Intravenous Bisphosphonate-Related Osteonecrosis of the Jaw: Bone Scintigraphy as an Early Indicator. Journal of Oral and Maxillofacial Surgery. 2009;**67**(7):1363-1372. DOI: 10.1016/j.joms.2009.03.005

[31] Hong CM et al. Implications of three-phase bone scintigraphy for the diagnosis of bisphosphonate-related osteonecrosis of the jaw. Nuclear Medicine and Molecular Imaging. 2012;**46**(3):162-168. DOI: 10.1007/s13139-012-0144-x

[32] Zhang L, He Q, Li W, Zhang R. The value of 99mTc-methylene diphosphonate single photon emission computed tomography/computed tomography in diagnosis of fibrous dysplasia. BMC Medical Imaging. 24 July 2017;**17**(1):46. DOI: 10.1186/s12880-017-0218-4

[33] Söderholm A-L et al. Bone scanning for evaluating mandibular bone extension of oral squamous cell carcinoma. Journal of Oral and Maxillofacial Surgery. 1990;**48**(3):252-257. DOI: 10.1016/0278-2391(90)90389-j

[34] Kletter K, Becherer A. FDG-PET in Der Onkologie. Der Radiologe. 1999;**39**(7):600-609. DOI: 10.1007/s001170050556

[35] Rohde M et al. 18F-fluoro-deoxy-glucose-positron emission tomography/computed tomography in diagnosis of head and neck squamous cell carcinoma: A systematic review and meta-analysis. European Journal of Cancer. 2014;**50**(13):2271-2279. DOI: 10.1016/j.ejca.2014.05.015

[36] Carvalho AL et al. Trends in incidence and prognosis for head and neck cancer in the United States: A site-specific analysis of the SEER database. International Journal of Cancer. 2004;**114**(5):806-816. DOI: 10.1002/ijc.20740

[37] Cacicedo J et al. Should PET/CT be implemented in the routine imaging work-up of locally advanced head and neck squamous cell carcinoma? A prospective analysis. European Journal of Nuclear Medicine and Molecular Imaging. 2015;**42**(9):1378-1389. DOI: 10.1007/s00259-015-3071-0

[38] Scott AM et al. PET changes management and improves prognostic stratification in patients with head and neck cancer: Results of a multicenter prospective study. Journal of Nuclear Medicine. 2008;**49**(10):1593-1600. DOI: 10.2967/jnumed.108.053660

[39] Connell CA et al. Clinical impact of, and prognostic stratification by, F-18 FDG PET/CT in head and neck mucosal squamous cell carcinoma. Head & Neck. 2007;**29**(11):986-995. DOI: 10.1002/hed.20629

[40] Benouaich V et al. Relevance of functional imaging in dental implantology. Journal of Clinical and Experimental Dentistry. 1 October 2018;**10**(10):e1011-e1016. DOI: 10.4317/jced.54816

[41] Nieweg OE et al. The definition of a sentinel node. Annals of Surgical Oncology. 2001;**8**(6):538-541. DOI: 10.1007/s10434-001-0538-y

[42] Surasi DS et al. 99mTc-Tilmanocept: A novel molecular agent for lymphatic mapping and sentinel lymph node localization. Journal of Nuclear Medicine Technology. 2015;**43**(2):87-91. DOI: 10.2967/jnmt.115.155960

[43] Vera DR et al. [99mTc] MAG3-mannosyl-dextran: A receptor-binding radiopharmaceutical for sentinel node detection. Nuclear Medicine and Biology. 2001;**28**(5):493-498. DOI: 10.1016/s0969-8051(01)00218-9

[44] Lymphoseek Prescribing Information. Lymphoseek Website. 2013. Available from: http://lymphoseek.com/assets/pdfs/Lymphoseek%20Package%20Insert%20-%20October%202014.pdf [Accessed: 23 April 2015]

[45] Riese CGU et al. Validity of sentinel node biopsy in early oral and oropharyngeal carcinoma. Journal of Cranio-Maxillofacial Surgery. 2018;**46**(10):1748-1752. DOI: 10.1016/j.jcms.2018.07.021

[46] Sharma D et al. Sentinel lymph node biopsy: A new approach in the management of head and neck cancers. Sultan Qaboos University Medical Journal. 2017;**17**(1):e3-e10. DOI: 10.18295/squmj.2016.17.01.002 [Accessed: 22 April 2020]

Section 2

Surgical Management of Oral and Maxillofacial Lesions

Chapter 6

Review of Current Practice for Temporomandibular Joint Meniscopexy Surgery

Omar Sheikh, Matin Ali Madadian and Amanveer Benning

Abstract

Disc repositioning for temporomandibular joint dysfunction (TMD) is a known and established procedure. Indications for the surgery and outcomes vary. A review of the available literature on the indications, surgical technique, and outcomes of TMJ Meniscopexy as a means of management of temporomandibular joint disease was performed. This was carried out using PubMed, MEDLINE, Scopus, and Google Scholar and was limited to the past 11 years using key medical search terms relevant to the subject area while being consistent with our exclusion criteria. The search yielded a total of 23 articles containing 3 reviews, 6 technical notes, 11 retrospective studies, and 3 prospective studies. Multiple techniques were described in the literature including arthroscopic techniques (n = 4), open suturing techniques (n = 4), mini-anchor techniques (n = 9), and splint-assisted surgery (n = 1). Several variables were used to determine success including both qualitative and quantitative measures determined clinically, through MRI or via patient questionnaire. When considering various combinations of these functional outcomes, all studies showed a significant improvement post-operatively. This demonstrates the success of disc repositioning procedures as an option in certain cases of TMD. Although there is evidence to show improvement in functional outcomes associated with Meniscopexy as a means of TMD management, there remains to be a lack of high-level evidence to further support this.

Keywords: temporomandibular joint, meniscoplasty, meniscopexy, disc repositioning, temporomandibular joint dysfunction

1. Introduction

Temporomandibular joint dysfunction (TMD) is the most common cause of non-odontogenic pain in the oro-facial region, having a significant impact on quality of life [1].

TMD is a common term used to describe a range of disorders affecting the temporomandibular joint. TMD can affect the temporomandibular joint (TMJ), the jaw muscles, or both, TMD has also been associated with ear and neck pain. Patients demonstrate clinical signs such as pain from the TMJ, muscle pain, TMJ sounds including clicking and crepitus, restricted mouth opening and deviation on mouth opening or closing [2].

The Research Diagnostic Criteria for Temporomandibular Disorders (RDC/TMD) presented by Dworkin and LeResche in 1992 classified TMD patients according to their physical diagnosis (axis I) and pain-related disability and psychological status (axis II). Axis I is divided into three groups. Group I is muscle disorders, Group II disc displacements and Group III consists of joint disorders as seen in the box below [3] (**Table 1**, **Figure 1**).

Classification systems have been conceived to further classify and delineate the specific groups discussed above. The Wilkes classification is used to classify TMJ Internal Derangement (**Table 2**).

The causes of TMD are wide and varied due to the homogeneity demonstrated in the classification. They include a wide range of direct injuries, such as fractures of the mandibular condyle, systemic diseases, including as immune mediated arthritis, growth disturbances and tumours. Non-functional movements of the mandible such as bruxing and tooth-clenching are clinically correlated with a variety of jaw muscle symptoms and are associated with internal joint disk derangements. It has been postulated however that these behaviours are not established causes of TMD but may only be propagating factors [5].

Malocclusion, previously thought to be causative is no longer widely established as an important factor in TMD. It has also been demonstrated that orthodontic treatment neither increases nor decreases the chances of developing TMD [5].

Different approaches have been described for the management of TMD depending on severity and aetiology. Initial management is non-surgical. This can range from physical therapy, occlusal appliance therapy, drug therapies, intra-articular injections, diet alteration and life style adaptation. Studies have demonstrated 70–80% of cases can be treated successfully with non-surgical interventions [4, 6].

Occlusal splint therapy has been reported with success. Various types of splints exist with distinctive indications and functions. The stabilisation splint is widely used; it is a hard acrylic splint and provides a temporary and removable ideal occlusion. Affording an occlusion reduces atypical muscle activity and produces neuromuscular balance to the TMJ [7].

Occlusal modification was proposed as a treatment however meta-analysis showed no evidence that it was beneficial in the management of TMD. Physiotherapy has been shown to be beneficial for a select group of patients [6].

Should conservative management strategies prove unsuccessful they may be followed by surgical intervention. These include menisectomy, disc repositioning, condylotomy and joint replacement. These procedures are aggressive and invasive with risks and complications of their own. Arthocentsis is considered less invasive and refers to lavage of the upper joint space, hydraulic pressure and manipulation to liberate adhesions and improve motion. Another less invasive procedure, TMJ arthroscopy is widely undertaken [8].

A review of arthroscopy and arthrocentesis found no statistically significant difference between these interventions in terms of pain, however a statistically significant difference in favour of arthroscopy was discovered in maximum incisal opening. The review concluded that there is insufficient reliable evidence to either encourage or disprove the use of arthrocentesis for treating patients with TMD and that further high quality studies are needed before firm conclusions can be stated [9].

Disc repositioning as a treatment for internal derangement of the temporomandibular disc was first reported to have been performed by Annandale in 1887 [10]. However, it was not until Wilkes first described the nature of the temporomandibular joint (TMJ) in TMD using arthrography in 1987 that surgical procedures such as disc repositioning were accepted as a means of management [11]. Notably, McCarty and Farrar were first to describe a rationale and technique for arthroplasty and disc repositioning for internal derangement of the TMJ in 1988 [12]. Since then, there

Group I—Muscle disorders	Group II—Disc displacements	Group III—Joint disorders
Ia. Myofascial pain: • Report of pain or ache in the jaw, temples, face, preauricular area, or inside the ear at rest or during function. • Pain on palpation of temporalis, masseter, lateral pterygoid area • At least one of the painful sites must be on the same side as the complaint of pain.	**IIa. Disc displacement with reduction:** • Reciprocal clicking in TMJ (click on both vertical opening and closing, occurring at point 5 mm greater than interincisal distance on opening than closing and is eliminated on protrusive opening), reproducible on 2 out of 3 consecutive trials • Clicking in TMJ either opening or closing, reproducible on 2 out of 3 consecutive trials, • Click during lateral excursion or protrusion, reproducible on 2 out of 3 consecutive trials.	**IIIa. Arthralgia:** • Pain in one or both joint sites (lateral pole and/or posterior attachment) during palpation • Pain in the region of the joint, pain in the joint during maximum unassisted opening, pain in the joint during assisted opening, and pain in the joint during lateral excursion • For a diagnosis of simple arthralgia, coarse crepitus must be absent.
Ib. Myofascial pain with limited opening: • As above with painless unassisted mandibular opening less than 40 mm. • Maximum assisted opening (passive stretch) less than 5 mm greater than painless unassisted opening.	**IIb. Disc displacement without reduction with limited opening:** • History of significant limitation in opening; • Maximum unassisted opening less than 35 mm; • Passive stretch increases opening by less than 4 mm over maximum unassisted opening • Contralateral excursion less than 7 mm and/or uncorrected deviation to ipsilateral side on opening • Absence of joint sound or presence of joint sounds not meeting criteria for disc displacement with reduction.	**IIIb. Osteoarthritis of the TMJ:** • Arthralgia as defined in IIIa; • Either coarse crepitus in the joint or radiologic signs of arthrosis.
	IIc. Disc displacement without reduction, without limited opening: • History of significant limitation of mandibular opening; • Maximum unassisted opening greater than 35 mm • Passive stretch increases opening by greater than 5 mm over maximum unassisted opening; • Contralateral excursion greater than 7 mm; • Presence of joint sounds not meeting criteria for disc displacement with reduction; • Where available, arthrography or magnetic resonance reveals disc displacement without reduction.	**IIIc. Osteoarthrosis of the TMJ:** • Absence of all signs of arthralgia; • Either coarse crepitus in the joint or radiologic signs of arthrosis.

Table 1.
RDC/TMD criteria for axis I diagnoses [3].

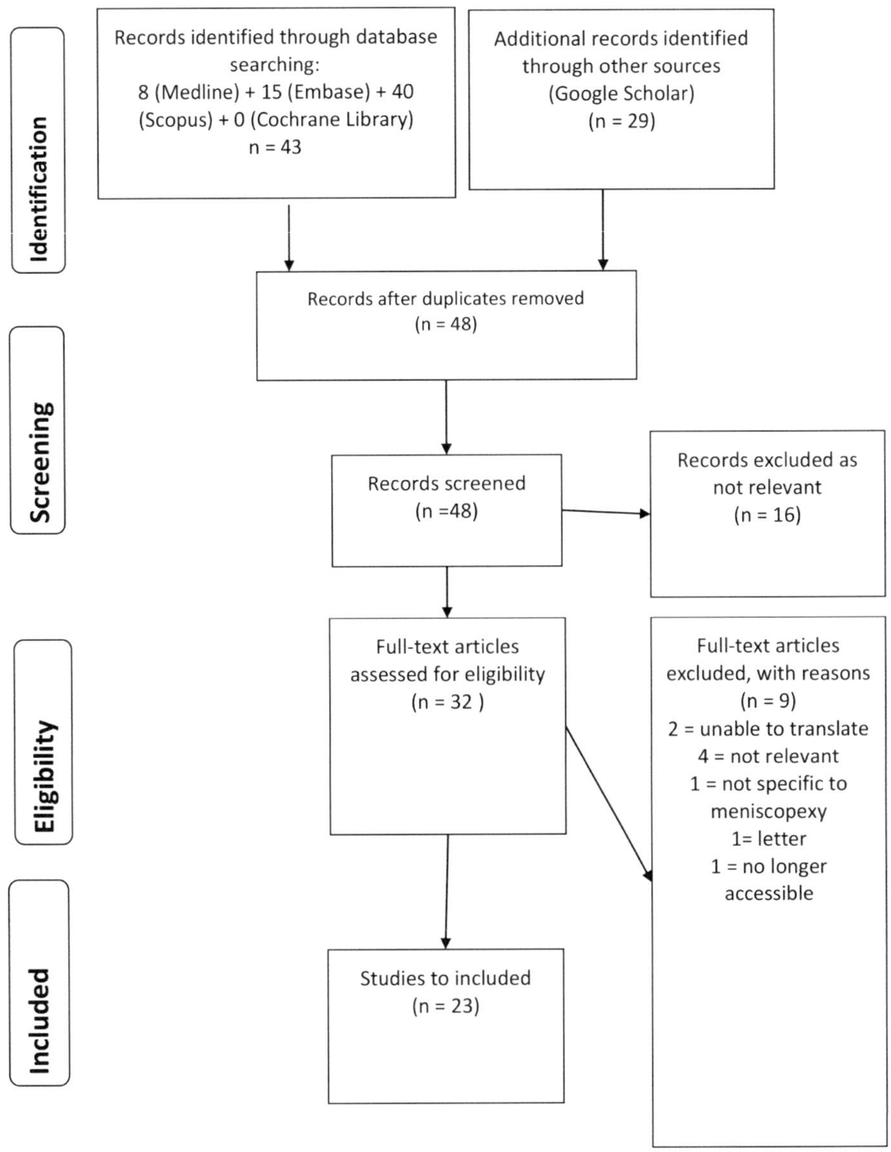

Figure 1.
PRISMA flow diagram, illustrating method by which screening of articles was undertaken.

have been multiple variations and modifications in technique that have been proposed by surgeons, each in an attempt to improve outcome [13]. Examples of such innovations are the introduction of orthopaedic suture anchors to with the hope of stabilising the disk more reliably and the advent of arthroscopy as an approach to repositioning the disc [14, 15].

The authors aim to look at current practice for meniscopexy, give an overview of the different TMJ articular disc repositioning techniques described as well as analysing clinical studies to establish their success by looking at measured functional outcomes. This enables us to scrutinise different approaches allowing us to conclude as to whether Meniscopexy remains to be a viable treatment modality in the management of TMD.

Stage	Clinical	Imaging	Surgical
I Early	Painless clicking. No restricted motion	Slightly forward disc, reducing. Normal osseous contours	Normal disc form. Slight anterior displacement. Passive incoordination (clicking)
II Early/Intermediate	Occasional painful clicking. Intermittent locking. Headaches	Slightly forward disc, reducing. Early disc deformity. Normal osseous contours	Anterior disc displacement. Thickened disc
III Intermediate	Frequent pain. Joint tenderness, headaches. Locking. Restricted motion. Painful chewing	Anterior disc displacement. Reducing early progressing to non-reducing late. Moderate to marked disc thickening. Normal osseous contours	Disc deformed and displaced. Variable adhesions. No bone changes
IV Intermediate/Late	Chronic pain, headache. Restricted motion	Anterior disc displacement non-reducing. Marked disc thickening. Abnormal bone contours	Degenerative remodelling of bony surfaces. Osteophtyes. Adhesions. Deformed disc without perforation
V Late	Variable pain. Joint crepitus. Painful function	Anterior disc displacement non-reducing with perforation and gross disc deformity. Degenerative osseous changes	Gross degenerative changes of disc and hard tissue. Perforation and multiple adhesions

Table 2.
The Wilkes classification [4].

2. Methods

Evidence was searched, using the Ovid Medline, Embase, Scopus and Cochrane Library medical databases. A literature search was carried out, in accordance with Prisma guidelines, on the PubMed/MEDLINE database as well as SCOPUS, Embase, Cochrane library medical databases and Google Scholar using key medical subject headings (MeSH) relevant to TMJ meniscopexy restricted to the past 11 years from the time of writing of this paper (**Table 3**).

The Key Terms we used included:

- Temporomandibular joint disorders
- TMD
- Temporomandibular joint
- TMJ
- Meniscopexy/Discopexy

Type	No. of Articles (%)
Review	3 (13)
Technical Note	6 (26)
Retrospective	12 (52)
Prospective	2 (9)

Table 3.
Articles found within literature search classified by type (published between 28/10/2008 and 28/10/2019).

- Meniscoplasty
- Disc Repositioning

We further scrutinised the list of papers using our inclusion criteria (below) to yield 23 relevant papers.

Inclusion criteria:

- Articles must be directly relevant to the to be evaluated
- Articles must be peer-reviewed
- Articles must be written in English
- Articles must be less than 11 years old (i.e., all articles published after 28/10/2008)
- Quantitative and Qualitative studies can be included

Excluded papers were patents, letters, articles not pertaining to meniscopexy treatment, articles not in the English language and those outside the stated timeline.

Of the 23 papers, we found 3 review articles, 12 retrospective studies, 2 prospective studies and 6 technical notes.

3. Methods

3.1 Indications for disc repositioning

Meniscopexy has been indicated in cases of anterior displacement of the TMJ articular disc without reduction, in an effort to slow progression to more advanced TMJ-related symptoms [16]. There are, however, a range of various surgical techniques that may be employed for TMD management, thus it is important to delineate where meniscopexy may be used in preference to these. Disc repositioning is favoured in patients who have not responded to initial non-surgical treatment [17] or diagnostic arthroscopy/arthrocentesis [18].

Studies have also attempted to identify causes of TMD that may have a more favourable surgical outcome with meniscopexy. One prospective cohort study looked at the stage of internal derangement of the articular disc according to the Wilkes classification as a factor in determining success using Meniscopexy in management. Patients had previously undergone both conservative and primary arthroscopic treatment with lysis and lavage of the superior joint space. Patients were classified into two groups, Wilkes Stages II and III and Wilkes Stages IV and

V and underwent arthroscopic disc repositioning surgery to reduce and fix the articular disc. The primary successful outcome was determined by absence of pain at 12 months postoperatively. The study found an 86.7% success rate for the Wilkes II/III group in comparison to 25% for the Wilkes IV/V group [18].

This suggests meniscopexy as being an effective means of management for earlier stages of internal derangement, but less successful with increasing degenerative changes of the TMJ. A literature review of discectomy versus preservation of the articular disc evaluated current evidence to determine a rationale for meniscopexy versus removal/replacement of the disc. Adequate remaining anatomy and mobility of the disc, with minimal damage or perforation was key to the decision to preserve [19, 20].

Surgical management of disc displacement without reduction arising acutely following facial trauma without condylar fracture where no TMJ symptoms existed prior to the event was evaluated. Evidence suggests that there is a more rapid progression of disease following acute displacement. There is a much weaker response to conservative treatment and greater chance of developing osteoarthiritis or even ankylosis of the joint, with fast degeneration of the condyle within the first 3 months. Such adverse degenerative changes in some patients would justify surgical intervention at an earlier stage rather than prolonged conservative treatment as first line management where necessary. Eight8 patients were offered disc repositioning surgery and seven total joint replacement following rapid onset of end-stage disease. The study observed patients following trauma, after both conservative treatment and surgery. All patients demonstrated limited maximum interincisal opening (MIO) and deterioration of the condyle as seen on MRI following initial conservative treatment, with significant improvement in MIO post-operatively [21].

Studies like this are useful in demonstrating the place for meniscopexy within the surgical armamentarium when managing TMDs. They give an appreciation where the procedure is most effective and can be indicated as a first line of approach. From the literature search there are no studies available that investigate the efficacy of meniscopexy over other techniques at various stages of disease. More data is required to inform surgeons of circumstances where meniscopexy has the best outcome.

3.2 Surgical technique

There are multiple surgical approaches described in the literature to TMJ articular disc repositioning, which can be broadly classified into three areas:

- Meniscopexy through an open incision or arthrotomy (described in 4 articles within our search) [16, 19, 22, 23]

- Meniscopexy with the use of suture anchors or mini-anchors to aid disc fixation (described in 10 articles within our search) [13, 15, 24–31]

- Arthroscopic meniscopexy (described in 4 articles within our search) [3, 14, 17, 32]

Disc repositioning techniques first developed, such as that initially described by McCarty and Farrar in 1988, rely on an endaural open incision to access the TMJ, which remains to be the approach of choice for many surgeons. Dissection is carried out to access the disc and is released anteriorly, repositioned and subsequently sutured, either to the capsule or auricular cartilage. This technique is favoured by many due to its relative ease, providing a better view of the disc and its attachments, making the anterior release and suturing of the disc more predictable, compared to arthroscopic surgery [16].

Modifications of this technique have been introduced, with the use of mini suture anchors screwed into the condyle, in the hope of achieving better long-term fixation and stability of the reduced disc. A variety of orthopaedic suture anchors have been used for this purpose, most commonly the Mitek [29] and Arthrex mini-anchors [15], however alternatives have also demonstrated success, such as one study that reports the use of orthodontic mini-screws [24]. Such techniques aim to offer a predictable long-term result, however, may not be most appropriate where it is difficult to insert a screw into the condyle, such as in the small, resorbed or osteoporotic condyle [16].

Arthroscopic repositioning of the disc and suturing provides an alternative to procedures involving an open incision. Arthroscopy is a more minimally invasive approach, permitting the selective operation on articular disc without causing damage to the other tissues of the TMJ, as well as reducing risk of iatrogenic facial nerve injury which can be associated with open surgery (arthrotomy). Surgically, this involves the creation of three portals, one for the arthroscope and two for instrumentation permitting the passing of a suture through the disc. This technique, despite its conservative nature, is mainly limited by its technical difficulty, and is best performed by an experienced surgeon to ensure a long-term stable outcome [16, 17, 32].

One article also reported the use of a modified meniscopexy technique, whereby a splint was used by patients for a period before surgery, opening the joint space. An anterior-repositioning splint was during the surgical procedure to place the mandible into an ideal relationship with the maxilla. The disc is finally repositioned and sutured anteriorly and laterally to the capsular ligament using an open preauricular approach. Patients then wear the splint postoperatively which is gradually made smaller and narrower, slowly reducing the joint space to its normal anatomical size with the aim of reducing displacement or relapse of the disc repositioning [22].

3.3 Outcome variables

Several outcome variables were used as measures post-surgery. These included maximal interincisal opening (MIO), post-operative pain using the visual analogue scale (VAS) or questionnaire, changes in diet consistency, mandibular range of motion, joint clicking (including other noises), the use of medications, joint loading signs, MRI to evaluate disc position, disc rupture, and muscular pain.

3.3.1 Maximal Interincisal opening (MIO)

MIO is the measurement of the distance between the incisal edges of maxillary central incisors to mandibular central incisors at maximum mouth opening. During anterior disc displacement, mandibular opening becomes limited, thus corrective meniscopexy should increase mouth opening in successful cases allowing MIO to be an indicator for success (**Table 4**).

When comparing the different techniques used in the studies, the greatest increase in mean MIO was seen for patients who had undergone arthrotomy using Mitek mini-anchors compared to arthroscopic techniques [17, 18, 21, 26, 28]. However, it should be noted that the severity of TMD within the patient cohorts is likely to differ, with higher Wilkes' classifications having further disc degeneration and thus limited mouth opening. Further to this, cohort size has implications on reliability of the results, with smaller cohorts being less reliable to compare surgical techniques based on outcomes. Rajkumar et al. found that MIO increased most significantly, in patients with disc displacement without reduction (DDwoR), within the first month after surgery, with significantly smaller increases seen up to 6 months post-operatively. Although it is difficult to compare between these studies

Name of study	Technique	Number of patients	Preoperative MIO mean (mm)	Postoperative MIO mean (mm)	Follow-up period (time post-op)
He et al. [21]	Disc repositioning/ Total joint replacement	8/7	19.8	33.9	Not specified
McCain et al. [18]	Arthroscopic suture meniscopexy	32	30.0	37.9	12 months
Ruiz Valero et al. [28]	Open Meniscopexy using Mitek anchors	50	23.5	38.3	Not specified
Goizueta Adame et al. [17]	Arthroscopic Meniscopexy using posterior double pass suture	16	31.1	39.9	12 months
Göçmen et al. [26]	Open Meniscopexy using Mitek anchors	7	22.8	31.5	12 months
Rajkumar et al. [24]	Open Meniscopexy with orthodontic anchors	3 patients with DDwoR*	25.6	35.0 39.6	1 month 6 months

DDwoR, disc displacement without reduction.

Table 4.
Pre-operative and post-operative mouth opening.

due to differing techniques used and other difference in key variables, similar trends can be seen from the values provided, highlighting the importance of correct disc position in mechanical action of the mandible.

3.3.2 Pain

Pain can be used as a subjective measure of surgical outcomes. Within the studies we looked at, there were three methods of measuring pain: using a questionnaire to give a pain score out of 10, using the Visual Analogue Scale (VAS) or by reporting the percentage of patients with pain pre and post operatively. These have been summarised in the table as average values within the patient cohorts (**Table 5**).

Overall, all studies showed an improvement in pain scores on follow up. The VAS was the most commonly used measure of quantifying pain improvement post-operatively. This can be said to be due to its relative simplicity and quantitative nature. However, there has been debate with regards to its validity. Patients may report pain with a certain degree of bias and also may not be able to report pain relief reliably owing to difficulties in recalling previous pain experiences, hence quantitative comparison is challenging [33]. Some studies looked at the simple absence/presence of pain: Ruiz Valero et al. demonstrated a significantly smaller number of patients presenting with painful TMJ symptoms 12 months post-operatively (pre-100%, post-8%). McCain et al. also looked at pain medication use among patients at pre-operative assessment (15/32 patients) and at last visit (6/32) as a secondary

Study	Surgical technique	No. of patients in cohort	Pre-op pain	Post-op pain	Follow-up period (time post-op)
McCain et al. [18]	Arthroscopic suture Meniscopexy	32	VAS score for joint function* 41.9	VAS score for joint function* 71.5	Not specified
Ruiz Valero et al. [28]	Open Meniscopexy with Mitek anchors	50	100% of patients	8% of patients	12 months
Sheikh et al. [22]	Splint assisted Meniscopexy	30	See separate table below	See Separate table below	8.5 years
Abramowicz et al. [23]	Not specified	18	9/10	1.3/10	20 years
Goizueta Adame et al. [17]	Arthroscopic Meniscopexy using posterior double pass suture	16	VAS score 7.6	VAS score 0.9	12 months
Sharma et al. [19]	Open Meniscopexy using Suture	10	Not specified	100% "Pain relief"	12 months
Göçmen et al. [26]	Open Meniscopexy with Mitek anchors	7	VAS Score 7.9	VAS score 0.6	12 months
Rajkumar et al. [24]	Open Meniscopexy with orthodontic anchors	10	Not specified	3.5	6 months

**This paper only presented scores for successful surgeries. Visual analogue scale in this paper ranged from 0 to 100 rather than 0 to –10, 0 indicating maximum pain and 100 no pain.*

Table 5.
Pre-operative and post-operative pain.

outcome variable. The subjective nature of pain presents difficulty when data gathering techniques are employed. Furthermore, only two articles measuring pain as an outcome variable in our search followed-up patients for more than 12 months [22, 23]. More studies are needed to look into more long-term data as a measure of success, especially with concerns of patients going on to develop secondary joint diseases in the long-term following disc-repositioning procedures [34]. Also, more sensitive means of pain measurement can be considered to establish pain relief post-operatively, if this is to be used as a primary outcome variable, such as the McGill pain questionnaire [35].

Sheikh et al. investigated pain using a different method. They asked patients about the frequency of pain compared to the severity as a measure of outcomes and found improvements from constant pain to rare and no pain. The table illustrates the distribution of pain frequency pre and post operatively [22] (**Table 6**).

This study looked at the pre and post-operative frequency of pain in 30 patients at a mean of 8.5 years post-op. Although the data illustrates a clear reduction in the frequency of pain within the cohort of patients, it would have been further enhanced by quantitative measures of frequency (e.g. pain occurring between 5 and 10 times per day, etc.). Currently, the interpretation of the terms used to describe pain by patients remains subjective. Further to this, if more data points were collected throughout the post-op period, the course of recovery could be monitored. Nevertheless, frequency of pain remains to be an interesting and useful alternative when measuring pain.

Frequency of pain	Pre-operatively (% of patients)	Post-operatively (% of patients)
Constant	66.67	3.33
Moderate	10	6.67
Occasionally	6.67	33.33
Rare	10	33.33
None	6.67	23.33

Table 6.
Pre-operative and post-operative pain distribution.

3.4 Mandibular range of motion

Arguably this is one of the most important outcomes as a patient's quality of life is greatly determined by this (ability to speak and chew). Goizueta Adame et al. specifically used lateral movements of the mandible as an outcome variable. They found on average in a cohort of 16 patients, the average lateral movement increased from 3.9 mm pre-op to 10.3 mm post-op [17].

Moreover, within the cohort patients looked into by Rajkumar et al., three patients had disc displacement without reduction and their lateral mandibular movements were recorded pre-op and at 6 months post-op. The pre-op average was 1.67 mm increasing to 4.67 mm at 6 months. However, this small patient size cannot be used to determine trends within the data. Further to this, other mandibular movements such as protrusion and retrusion could have been recorded over the long term throughout the studies, in order to create a more complete picture of mandibular function [24].

3.5 Evaluation of disc position using MRI post-operatively

Four studies used MRI evaluation post-operatively looking at disc positioning and condylar changes, as a means to qualify the effectiveness of TMJ meniscopexy procedures.

Zhang et al. conducted a study with 81 patients with internal derangement of the articular disc, ranging from Wilkes III to V that underwent meniscopexy using bone anchors for fixation. MRI was performed 1–7 days post-operatively to evaluate the position of the disc as poor (none or only reposition in one sagittal plane), good (reposition in two2 sagittal planes) or excellent (reposition in three sagittal planes). They termed a successful outcome as good or better and found that 77 patients were excellent, 1 patient had good outcome and 3 patients had poor outcomes, suggesting a 96.3% success rate using bone anchors in arthrotomy [27].

Comparable results are seen in a study of 764 joints treated with an arthroscopic disc repositioning technique, with 729/764 joints deemed as having an excellent outcome [32]. In this particular study however, the specific suture technique was not described, making comparison difficult.

Such data proves that various techniques can be effectively used to reposition the disc accurately into its anatomic position. However, the efficacy of the techniques described can be attributed to the skill of the operator, and such results may not be reproducible universally. Furthermore, while this data gives a good indication of how well the disc is reduced immediately post-operatively, more information regarding long-term relapse would be useful to determine success. The study also gives no mention of post-operative pain or function. Outcomes that are more important to patients than knowing their disc is in the correct position.

Rajkumar et al. conducted MRI assessment at 6 months for 10 patients managed with meniscopexy with orthodontic mini-screws, finding stable positioning of the disc and lack of progression of arthritic changes of the condyle on evaluation [24]. Zhou et al. when using MRI scans to follow up patients post-operatively found 4.7% of patients relapsed with anterior disc displacement. Of the 149 patients, 5 relapsed after 1 year and 2 after 2 years [25]. However, further studies investigating the long-term follow up of all cases is required to accurately ascertain incidence of relapse.

Other outcomes such as reduction in joint noises, increase in diet consistency, muscle pain and joint loading signs were also looked at in a few isolated studies as a means to assess the success of surgery. However, there were not enough studies available to effectively use these to determine outcomes.

4. Discussion

From the results of our search it is reasonable to conclude that there is data to support the efficacy of meniscopexy for the management of temporomandibular joint dysfuction. Studies evaluating various techniques of articular disc repositioning demonstrated a successful outcome in the majority of cases, with little evidence to prove otherwise. However, there are certain limitations present in the literature available:

- There is a lack of high-level evidence to evaluate outcomes.
- There is limited evidence looking at long-term follow up of patients who have received meniscopexy.
- No study currently compares the efficacy of meniscopexy directly relative to other surgical techniques available (*e.g.* arthroscopy/arthrocentesis or total joint replacement) to establish its superiority in similar groups of patients.
- There is a lack of consistency in outcome variables evaluated and method in which these were determined, as well as surgical techniques used between papers. Some studies did not describe technique used. Therefore, it is difficult to compare and collate the results of various studies.
- Many of the procedures described are sensitive techniques, and therefore results may not necessarily be reproducible across centres or among different operators.

4.1 Levels of evidence

According to the *Oxford Centre for Evidence-Based Medicine* 2011 guidelines on levels of evidence in healthcare research [36], the highest levels of evidence consist of systematic reviews of randomised trials *(Level I)* or randomised trials or observational studies with dramatic effect *(Level II)*. The difficulty in conducting randomised, controlled trials prospectively to evaluate outcomes of surgery in this field limit the quality and certainty of conclusions that can be made with regards to effectiveness.

4.2 Follow-up

Our literature search only yielded 2 articles following up patients for more than 12 months after having received disc repositioning surgery, neither of which was conducted prospectively [22, 23]. Concerns exist with regard to long-term outlook of this surgery, specifically incidence of relapse, reoccurrence of symptoms and secondary joint disease [34, 37]. Well-designed, prospective studies of patients receiving meniscopexy with prolonged follow-up are required to address these concerns.

4.3 Comparison to other techniques

No one surgical technique in the management of advanced TMD seems to predominate, with multiple options described in the literature. Where procedures such as arthrocentesis of the joint space are successful in the management of internal derangement, the role of disc position in the pathology of TMD should be questioned [37]. Ribeiro et al. [38] found articular disc displacement without symptoms to be a common occurrence in the general population (34% of subjects) when conducting an MRI study of 56 asymptomatic volunteers. Other authors [39, 40] have also questioned the role of disc position in TMJ pathology, arguing that pathological changes such as synovitis, osteoarthritis and adhesions to be the causative agents of symptoms, which should be treated separately.

However, in instances where there is no response to other treatment, there seems to be benefit in meniscopexy. This suggests there may still be a place for disc mobilisation, with many patients showing immediate improvement in mechanical function potentially leading to better regeneration of the tissues [17].

Other surgeries performed such as discectomy, joint replacement procedures and various other arthrotomies may also be beneficial in particular circumstances [20]. Since a single procedure has not yet been identified as being preferable in all instances of TMD, the role of the surgeon then becomes to identify the modality which will achieve the best outcome on a case-by-case basis.

To establish the place of meniscopexy relative to other techniques at the operator's disposal research is required comparing surgical modalities. Despite positive findings no study exists offering a direct comparison between repositioning the disc and alternative procedures.

4.4 Technical limitations

A number of different approaches are described to reposition the articular disc, some of which are more technically demanding. No study was found directly comparing the efficacy of different techniques. This is also hard to determine since the efficacy of certain techniques will largely depend on the skill of the operator [13]. For instance, excellent outcomes have been reported with arthroscopic disc repositioning and suturing techniques [32]. However, such results may not be reproducible due to this technically demanding technique, resulting in data that is not universally acceptable [16].

5. Conclusion

Despite the fact that an increasingly greater proportion of TMD is being managed conservatively and minimally invasively, there remains a place for surgical procedures in refractory cases. There is evidence in the literature to suggest meniscopexy is an effective procedure in the management of some instances of TMD, however high-level evidence is lacking. Outcome variables between papers varied, making comparison difficult. In addition, it is apparent that many other techniques are available at a surgeon's disposal, many of which may be more effective than attempts to reposition the disc. Therefore, case selection is vital when deciding to use meniscopexy as a primary means of management, something which is currently largely based on clinical experience. More research into the pathological processes underlying TMD is required to allow surgeons to make more justified and informed decisions on appropriate means of management for each individual case.

Author details

Omar Sheikh*, Matin Ali Madadian and Amanveer Benning
Kings College Hospital, London, United Kingdom

*Address all correspondence to: osheikh@nhs.net

References

[1] Durham J, Newton-John TRO, Zakrzewska JM. Temporomandibular disorders. BMJ. 2015;**350**:h1154

[2] Leresche L. Epidemiology of temporomandibular disorders: Implications for the investigation of etiologic factors. Critical Reviews in Oral Biology and Medicine. 1997;**8**: 291-305

[3] Dworkin SF, Leresche L. Research diagnostic criteria for temporomandibular disorders: Review, criteria, examinations and specifications, critique. Journal of Craniomandibular Disord Facial Oral Pain. 1992;**6**:301-355

[4] Ahmed N, Sidebottom AJ. The role arthroscopy and arthrocentesis in TMJ management. Face Mouth & Jaw Surgery: International Trainee Journal of Oral & Maxillofacial Surgery. 2012;**2**:1-3

[5] Tanaka E, Detamore MS, Mercuri LG. Degenerative disorders of the temporomandibular joint: Etiology, diagnosis and treatment. Journal of Dental Research. 2008;**87**:296-307

[6] Rajapakse S, Ahmed N, Sidebottom AJ. Current thinking about the management of dysfunction of the temporomandibular joint: A review. The British Journal of Oral & Maxillofacial Surgery. 2017;**55**(4):351-356. DOI: 10.1016/j.bjoms.2016.06.027

[7] Davies SJ, Gray RJ. The pattern of splint usage in a®the management of two common temporomandibular disorders. Part II: The stabilisation splint in the treatment of pain dysfunction syndrome. British Dental Journal. 1997;**183**(7):247-251

[8] Nitzan DW, Dolwick MF, Martinez GA. Temporomandibular joint arthrocentesis: A simplified treatment for severe, limited mouth opening. Journal of Oral and Maxillofacial Surgery. 1991;**49**(11):1163-1167

[9] Guo C, Shi Z, Revington P. Arthrocentesis and lavage for treating temporomandibular joint disorders. Cochrane Database of Systematic Reviews. 2009;(Issue 4):CD004973. DOI: 10.1002/14651858.CD004973.pub2

[10] Annandale T. On displacement of the inter-articular cartilage of the lower jaw, and its treatment by operation. The Lancet. 1887;**129**(3313):411

[11] Wilkes CH. Arthrography of the temporomandibular joint in patients with the TMJ pain-dysfunction syndrome. Minnesota Medicine. 1978;**61**:645-652

[12] McCarty WL, Farrar WB. Surgery for internal derangements of the temporomandibular joint. Journal of Prosthetic Dentistry. 1979;**42**(2):191-196

[13] Gonçalves JR, Cassano DS, Rezende L, Wolford LM. Disc repositioning: Does it really work? Oral and Maxillofacial Surgery Clinics. 2015;**27**(1):85-107

[14] Yang C, Cai X, Chen M, Zhang S. New arthroscopic disc repositioning and suturing technique for treating an anteriorly displaced disc of the temporomandibular joint: Part I–technique introduction. International Journal of Oral and Maxillofacial Surgery. 2012;**41**(9):1058-1063

[15] Ryba FM, Ali A, Matthews NS. Temporomandibular joint meniscopexy using the Arthrex Ccorkscrew® mini anchor system: Technical note. British Journal of Oral and Maxillofacial Surgery. 2015;**53**(3):299-300

[16] He D, Yang C, Zhu H, Ellis E. Temporomandibular joint disc

repositioning by suturing through open incision: A technical note. Journal of Oral and Maxillofacial Surgery. 2018;**76**(5):948-954

[17] Goizueta Adame CC, Muñoz-Guerra MF. The posterior double pass suture in repositioning of the temporomandibular disc during arthroscopic surgery: A report of 16 cases. Journal of Cranio-Maxillo-Facial Surgery. 2012;**40**(1):86-91

[18] McCain JP, Hossameldin RH, Srouji S, Maher A. Arthroscopic discopexy is effective in managing temporomandibular joint internal derangement in patients with Wilkes stage II and III. Journal of Oral and Maxillofacial Surgery. 2015;**73**(3):391-401

[19] Sharma R, Sinha R, Menon PS. Meniscopexy for internal derangement of temporomandibular joint. J Maxillofac Oral Surg. 2010;**9**(3):261-265

[20] Renapurkar SK. Discectomy versus disc preservation for internal derangement of the temporomandibular joint. Oral and Maxillofacial Surgery Clinics of North America. 2018;**30**(3):329-333

[21] He D, Yang X, Wang F, Yang C, Dong M. Acute trauma induced disc displacement without reduction and its sequelae. Scientific Reports. 2016;**6**(1):32684

[22] Sheikh O, Logan G, Komath D, Grossman P, Ayliffe P. Splint-assisted disc plication surgery. Annali di Stomatologia. 2016;**7**(3):73

[23] Abramowicz S, Dolwick MF. 20-year follow-up study of disc repositioning surgery for temporomandibular joint internal derangement. Journal of Oral and Maxillofacial Surgery. 2010;**68**(2):239-242

[24] Rajkumar K, Roy Chowdhury SK, Sinha R. Clinical and MRI evaluation of orthodontic mini-screws for disc repositioning in internal derangement of TMJ: A prospective study. J Maxillofac Oral Surg. 2018;**17**(1):52-58

[25] Zhou Q, Zhu H, He D, Yang C, Song X, Ellis E. Modified temporomandibular joint disc repositioning with Miniscrew anchor: Part II-stability evaluation by magnetic resonance imaging. Journal of Oral and Maxillofacial Surgery. 2019;**77**(2):273-279

[26] Göçmen G, Varol A, Karatas B, Basa S. Evaluation of temporomandibular joint disc-repositioning surgery with Mitek mini anchors. National Journal of Maxillofacial Surgery. 2013;**4**(2):188-192

[27] Zhang S, Liu X, Yang X, Yang C, Chen M, Haddad MS, et al. Temporomandibular joint disc repositioning using bone anchors: An immediate post surgical evaluation by magnetic resonance imaging. BMC Musculoskeletal Disorders. 2010;**11**:262

[28] Ruiz Valero CA, Marroquin Morales CA, Jimenez Alvarez JA, Gomez Sarmiento JE, Vallejo A. Temporomandibular joint meniscopexy with Mitek mini anchors. Journal of Oral and Maxillofacial Surgery. 2011;**69**(11):2739-2745

[29] Rajkumar K, Mukhopadhyay P, Sinha R. Temporomandibular joint disc repositioning using an orthopedic suture anchor: A modified disc anchoring technique. Journal of Maxillofacial Oral Surgery. 2016;**15**(3):404-407

[30] Spallaccia F, Rivaroli A, Basile E, Cascone P. Disk repositioning surgery of the temporomandibular joint with bioabsorbable anchor. The Journal of Craniofacial Surgery. 2013;**24**(5):1792-1795

[31] He D, Yang C, Zhang S, Wilson JJ. Modified temporomandibular joint disc repositioning with miniscrew anchor: Part I--surgical technique. Journal of Oral and Maxillofacial Surgery. 2015;**73**(1):9

[32] Zhang S, Liu X, Yang C, Cai X, Chen M, Haddad MS, et al. New arthroscopic disc repositioning and suturing technique for treating internal derangement of the temporomandibular joint: Part II--magnetic resonance imaging evaluation. Journal of Oral and Maxillofacial Surgery. 2010;**68**(8):1813-1817

[33] Carlsson AM. Assessment of chronic pain. I. Aspects of the reliability and validity of the visual analogue scale. Pain. 1983;**16**(1):87-101

[34] Sidebottom AJ. Current thinking in temporomandibular joint management. The British Journal of Oral & Maxillofacial Surgery. 2009;**47**(2):91-94

[35] Melzack R. The McGill pain questionnaire: Major properties and scoring methods. Pain. 1975;**1**(3):277-299

[36] OCEBM Levels of Evidence Working Group. The Oxford 2011 Levels of Evidence. Oxford Centre for Evidence-Based Medicine. 2011. Availbale from: http://www.cebm.net/index.aspx?o=5653

[37] Dolwick MF. The role of temporomandibular joint surgery in the treatment of patients with internal derangement. Oral Surgery, Oral Medicine, Oral Pathology, Oral Radiology, and Endodontology. 1997;**83**(1):150-155

[38] Ribeiro RF, Tallents RH, Katzberg RW, Murphy WC, Moss ME, Magalhaes AC, et al. The prevalence of disc displacement in symptomatic and asymptomatic volunteers aged 6 to 25 years. Journal of Orofacial Pain. 1997;**11**(1):37-47

[39] Dolwick MF. Intra-articular disc displacement part I: Its questionable role in temporomandibular joint pathology. Journal of Oral and Maxillofacial Surgery. 1995;**53**(9):1069-1072

[40] Israel HA, Langevin C, Singer MD, Behrman DA. The relationship between Temporomandibular joint Synovitis and adhesions: Pathogenic mechanisms and clinical implications for surgical management. Journal of Oral and Maxillofacial Surgery. 2006;**64**(7):1066-1074

Chapter 7

Diagnosis and Management of Mandibular Condyle Fractures

Kasi Ganesh Sriraam and K. Rajendran Arun Vignesh

Abstract

In the maxillofacial region, mandibular condyle fracture accounts for about 10–40% of the trauma spectrum. This chapter deals with the etiology, classification, clinical features, diagnosis, and contemporary management of mandibular condyle fractures. Along with the regular management strategies, treatment protocols for geriatric and pediatric patients have also been discussed. The indications and contraindications of closed as well as open reduction and fixation of condyle fractures are analyzed in detail.

Keywords: mandible, condyle, trauma, clinical features, diagnosis, management, ORIF, closed reduction, edentulous, pediatric, complications

1. Introduction

Mandible is the second most commonly fractured after nasal bone, though it is the largest and strongest bone. Mandibular condyle fractures accounts for about 10–40% when compared to other anatomical sites of mandible [1]. The proportion of condylar fractures is higher in children than adults, and has been reported to account for 40–67% of mandibular fractures [2]. According to Widmark and Santler, condylar fracture is the most common fracture in the maxillofacial region [1]. Direct or indirect trauma can lead to fracture of the condyle; the degree of displacement depends on the direction and magnitude of the force. Falls, road traffic accident, sports injuries, work-related injuries and assault are frequently related to condylar fracture [3].

2. Anatomy

Condyle develops from Meckel's cartilage and it is intramembranous in ossification. The secretion of bone matrix directly within the connective tissue without any intermediate cartilage leads to bone formation. The condensation of mesenchyme just lateral to the Meckel's cartilage forms the primitive condyle.

Condyle is a knuckle like structure. It is a strong upward projection from the postero-superior part of the ramus. The condyle has a backward angulation of 15–33° to the frontal plane and is elliptical in shape. The condyle has an angulation of 145–160° at the region where it meets at the anterior ligament of foramen magnum on basion. The medio-lateral width is 15–20 mm and the antero-posterior width is 8–10 mm. The condyle has a roughened, bluntly pointed lateral pole and a rounded medial pole which extends from the plane of ramus. Superficial temporal artery, posterior tympanic artery, posterior deep temporal artery and transverse facial artery provides the arterial supply to the condyle. Venous drainage is by the corresponding tributaries. Nerve supply is from facial and auriculotemporal nerves. Lateral pterygoid muscle is attached at the pterygoid fovea which is helpful in protrusive and lateral excursive movements [4].

The bifurcation of facial nerve lies 1.5–2 cm away from the bony external auditory canal. The Temporal branch of the facial nerve lies 8–35 mm from the bony external auditory canal. The marginal mandibular branch of the facial nerve lies 1.2 cm away from the inferior border.

The anatomical variations between an adult and a pediatric condyle are given in **Table 1** (**Figures 1** and **2**).

Anatomical structure	Child	Adult
Cortical bone	Thin	Thick
Condylar neck	Broad	Thin
Articular surface	Thin	Thick
Capsule	Highly vascular	Less vascular

Table 1.
Differences between pediatric and adult condyle.

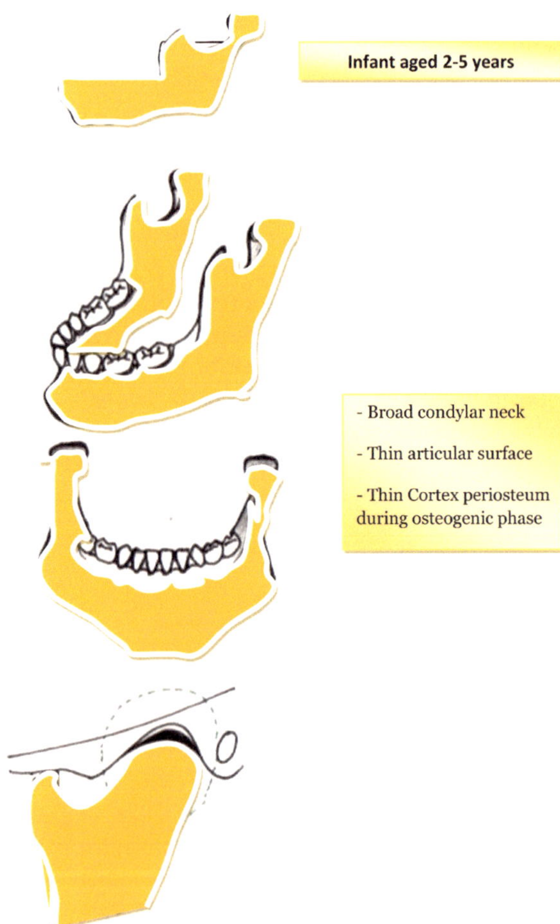

Figure 1.
Anatomy of Paediatric condyle.

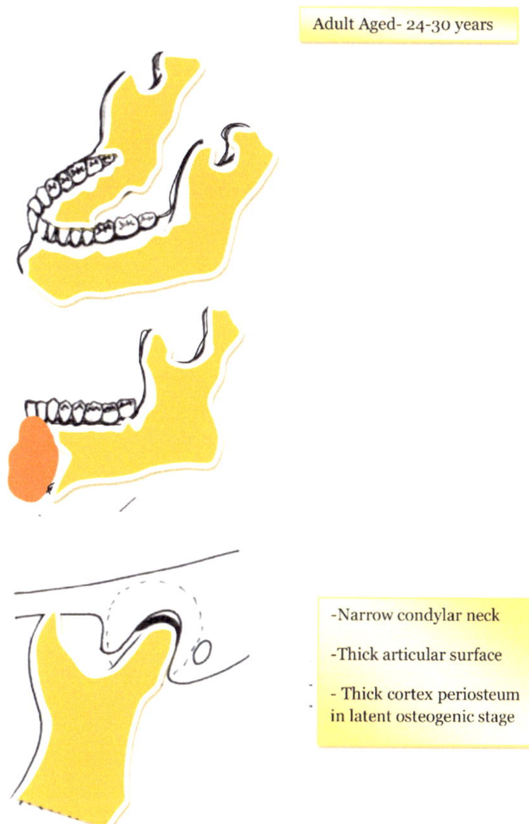

Figure 2.
Anatomy of adult condyle.

3. Biomechanics of injury (Hunting bow concept)

The Mandible resembles a Hunting bow which is weak at the ends and strong in the midline and the condyles are enclosed by the glenoid fossa. So any blow to the midline of the mandible can cause bilateral condylar fracture and any blow to the parasymphysis may cause a contralateral fracture. This is based on the impact of the force (**Figure 3**) [5].

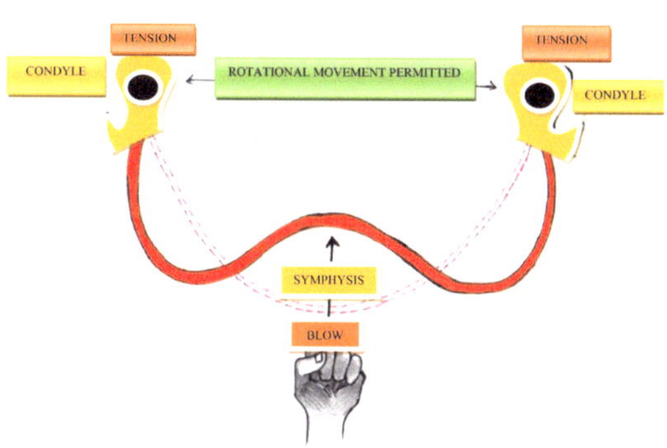

Figure 3.
Hunting bow concept.

The fracture of condyle following trauma to the chin is an example of contre-coup injury. This is commonly found in soldiers who remain standing for a long time and hence referred to as Parade ground/Guardsman fracture.

4. Classification of condylar fractures

Numerous classifications of condylar fractures are found in literature based on clinical and radiographic features.

4.1 Wassmund 1927

Based on:

a. Comminuted head fractures

b. Chip fractures

c. Condylar neck fractures
   i. Vertical neck fractures secondary to shearing
   ii. Transverse neck fractures secondary to bending
   iii. Oblique neck fractures caused by a combination/bending [6]

4.2 Wassmund 1934

Based on dislocated fractures of the condyle:
Type I: bony contact between the fractured fragments with 10–40° angulation of the condylar head.
Type II: bony contact between the fractured fragments with 50–90° angulation of the condylar head.
Type III: no bony contact with severe medial displacement [6].

4.3 Lindahl 1977

Based on the fracture location, deviation, and/or displacement and position of the condylar head within the articulating fossa:

- Sub condylar fracture: fracture line extends from the sigmoid notch to the posterior border of the mandible.

- Condylar neck fracture: fracture located below the level of condylar head at the condylar process.

- Condylar head fracture: fracture enclosed by the capsule of the temporomandibular joint (**Figure 4**)

1. Fracture level

   a. Condylar head

   b. Condylar neck

   c. Sub condylar/condylar base

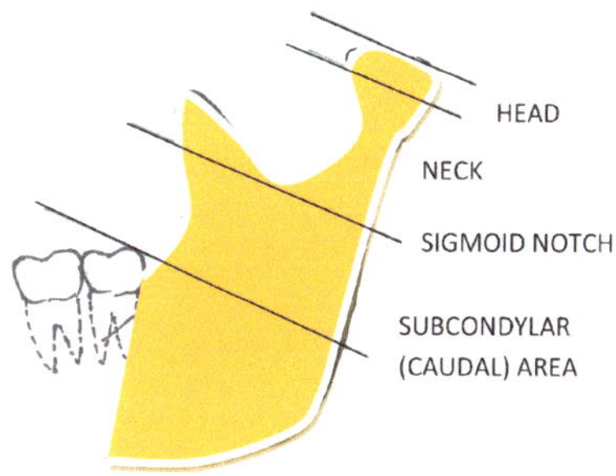

Figure 4.
Lindahl classification.

2. Deviation and displacement

   a. Medial overlapping with bending or deviation

   b. Lateral overlapping with bending or deviation

   c. No overlapping with bending or displacement

   d. No deviation or displacement

3. Relation between condylar head and fossa

   a. Absence of dislocation

   b. Mild dislocation

   c. Moderate dislocation

   d. Complete or severe dislocation

4. Condylar head fracture

   a. Horizontal

   b. Vertical

   c. Compression fracture [6]

4.4 Loukota 2005

This Classification described "Line A," which is a perpendicular line that extends from the deepest part of the coronoid notch to the posterior border of mandibular ramus.

- Diacapitular fracture: involves the articular surface and may extend outside the capsule of the temporomandibular joint

- Condylar neck: more than half of the fracture line is above line A

- Condylar base: more than half of the fracture line is below line A originating behind the mandibular foramen
- Minimal displacement: less than 10 mm of displacement or less than 2 mm of overlap by the bony edges or both [6]

4.5 The AO 2010

Based on:

- The first line parallels the posterior border of the mandible.
- The sigmoid notch line runs perpendicular to the first line at the deepest portion of the sigmoid notch.
- There is a line below the lateral pole of the condylar head that is also perpendicular to the first line.
- A line is drawn half way between the lateral pole line and the sigmoid notch line.
- A "high-neck" fracture is above this line, whereas a "low-neck" fracture is below [6].

4.6 Neff 2014

Based on the disc and condylar head:

- Condylar head: the condylar head reference line runs perpendicular to the posterior ramus below the lateral pole of the condylar head.
- Condylar neck: the sigmoid notch line running through the deepest point of the sigmoid notch perpendicular to the ramus line extending superiorly to the condylar head.
- Base of the condylar process: the sigmoid notch line running through the deepest point of the sigmoid notch perpendicular to the ramus line extending inferiorly [7].

4.7 Ying 2017

Classification of condylar head fracture based on vertical height of the ramus and disc displacement:

- Type A— no disc displacement or decrease in vertical height of the ramus
- Type B—disc displacement without decrease in vertical height of the ramus
- Type C—decrease in vertical height of the ramus with/without disc displacement [8]

5. Clinical examination

Condyle fractures are diagnosed with the help of both clinical and radiological assessment. Condylar fractures are most commonly missed on clinical examination. Extracapsular condylar fractures are frequent and may be associated with displacement of the condylar head. The condylar head may be in contact with the ramus or can be displaced laterally or medially. Anteromedial displacement is more common due to the pull of lateral pterygoid and weak medial capsule.

5.1 On inspection

a. Unilateral condylar fracture:

- Swelling over the temporomandibular joint, may be associated with hemorrhage from the external ear (due to laceration of external acoustic meatus by the violent impact of condyle on the skin).
- Proper examination with an autoscope/auriscope is essential to differentiate bleeding from external auditory canal and middle ear. Temporal bone may be accompanied by cerebrospinal fluid leak which is termed as otorrhea.
- Hematoma surrounding the fractured condyle
- Hematoma in the mastoid region called the Battle's sign
- If the condylar head is displaced medially, characteristic hollow in the region of condylar head can be observed once the edema subsides.
- Ear bleed will persist if the head of the condyle is impacted in the glenoid fossa.
- Deviation of mandible toward the side of fracture
- Decreased range of movements, pain and deviation toward the contra-lateral side while mouth opening.
- Gagging of occlusion on the ipsilateral side due to telescoping of fracture fragments on the contralateral side due to contraction of the masseter, temporalis and medial pterygoid and upward pull of the ramal segment (**Figure 5**)

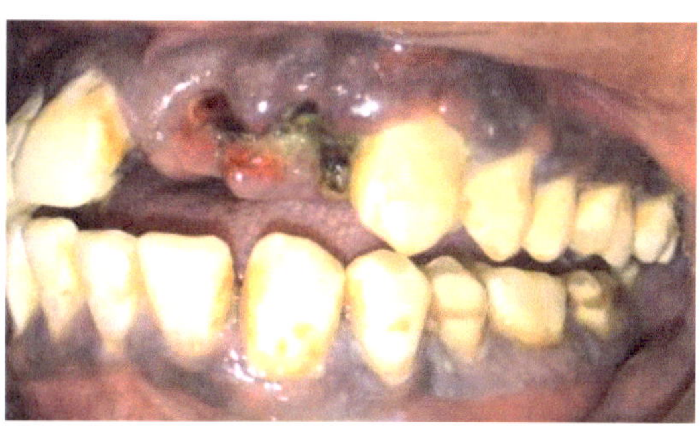

Figure 5.
Ipsilateral open bite.

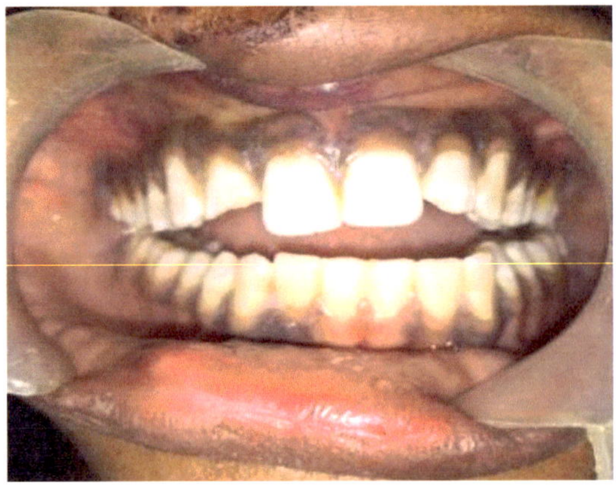

Figure 6.
Anterior open bite.

b. Bilateral condylar fracture:

- Overall mandibular movements are usually more restricted
- If the condyle is displaced bilaterally, shortening of ramus occurs resulting in derangement of occlusion
- Overriding of the fractured segments result in anterior open bite (**Figure 6**)
- Associated fracture of symphysis or para-symphysis can also be present; thus careful examination is mandatory (Contre-coupe fracture)

5.2 On palpation

- The condyles are palpated by standing in front of the patient. The little fingers are placed inside the external auditory canal and the patient is asked to open and close their mouth, by this method the position and movement of the condyles are determined.
- Tenderness over the condylar area
- Displacement of the condylar head within the external auditory meatus.
- Paresthesia of the lips may be present as the hemorrhage from the condylar region tracks across the base of skull and exerts pressure on the mandibular division of the trigeminal nerve as it emerges from the foramen ovale.

6. Radiographic assessment

Routine radiological investigations that aids in the diagnosis of condylar fracture are:

- Posteroanterior skull projection or Reverse Towne's (**Figure 7**)
- Oblique-lateral X-ray
- Orthopantomographic radiograph (**Figure 8**)

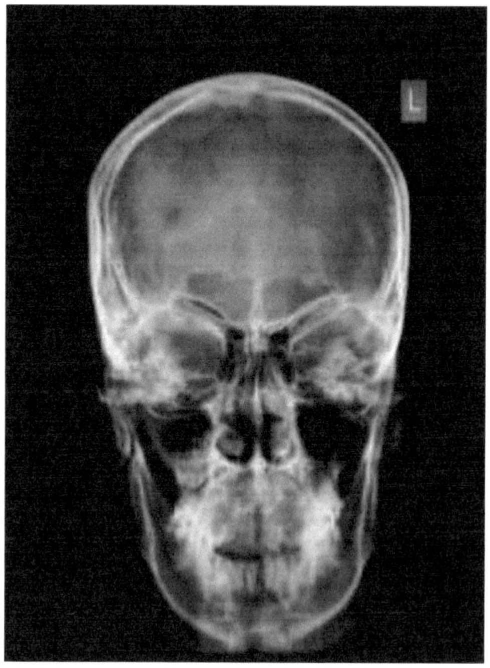

Figure 7.
Posterior anterior skull view.

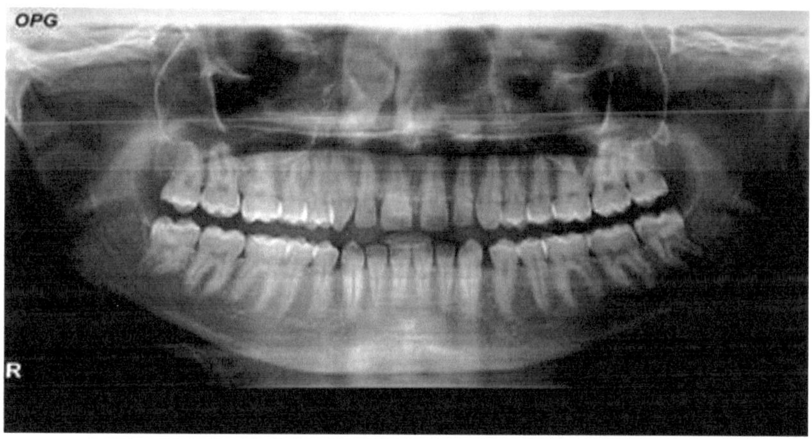

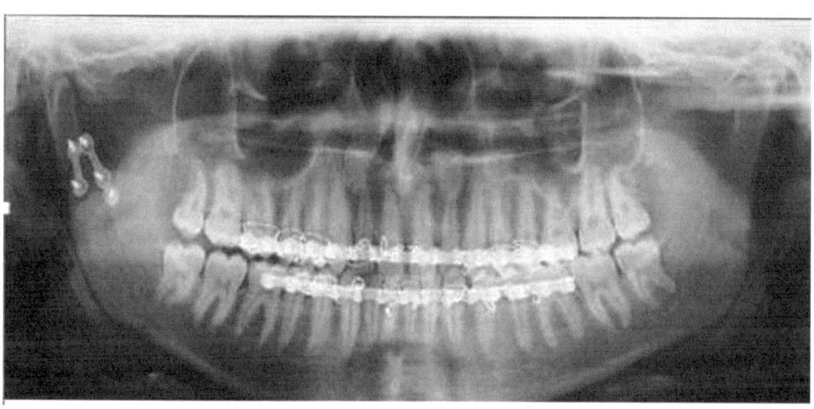

Figure 8.
Orthopantomogram.

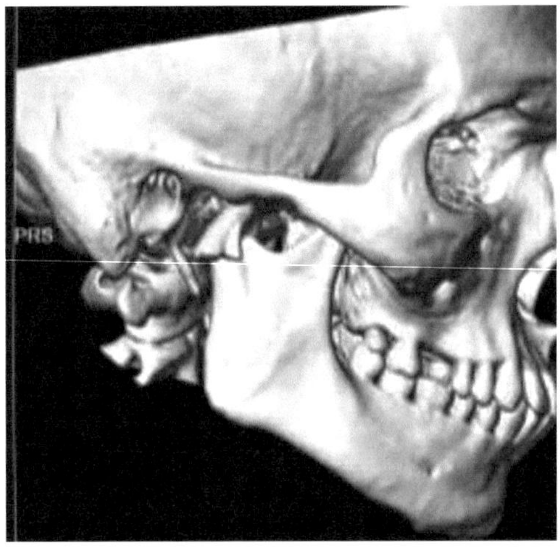

Figure 9.
Computed tomography.

- TMJ tomography
- Waters projection or Para nasal sinus view
- Clementschitsch view or occipital
- Nasal projection [9]

CT in all three planes, i.e., coronal, axial, and sagittal remains a gold standard for the diagnosis of mandibular condyle fractures. 3D CT provides better orientation of the fractured fragments in relation to the normal anatomic structures (**Figure 9**) [10].

Determining the degree of dislocation, relationship between the fractured fragments and the direction of dislocation remains a challenge in the diagnosis of mandibular condyle fractures. It may be difficult to ascertain position and rotation of the articular head of the condyle with the use of conventional imaging techniques. MRI may provide a better outlook in assessing both the hard tissue and soft tissue part of the condylar head. One must remember that re-establishing only the bony component of the joint is not sufficient and the soft tissue anatomy (Articular disc) must also be restored to achieve satisfactory functional outcomes [11].

7. Management of condylar fractures

Aims of treatment includes

1. Restoration of form
2. Restoration of function

This is achieved by proper repositioning and immobilization of the fractured fragments.

Treatment options for mandibular condyle fractures can be divided into conservative treatment and surgical management [9].

8. Conservative treatment of condylar fractures

Conservative therapy remained the primary mode of treatment of mandibular condyle fracture for many years. This is now overshadowed by surgical therapy due to increase in surgical expertise and the advent of new technological advances in both instrumentation and radiological diagnosis. But there exist certain scenarios where conservative treatment is preferred.

In closed reduction achievement of good occlusal relationship acts as the guidance for proper reduction. The upper and lower jaws are fixed together in occlusal relationship by means of intermaxillary fixation or maxillomandibular fixation done using wires or splints. The wires that pass through the embrasure space of the adjacent teeth of the same arch are called interdental wires. These are later engaged during intermaxillary wiring.

Various modalities of intermaxillary fixation used commonly for condylar fracture are:

1. Wiring:

- Ivy loop wiring
- Continuous ivy loop wiring
- Gilmer wiring

2. Arch bars:

- Erich's arch bar

3. Splints:

- Cap splint in pediatric patients
- Gunning splints in edentulous patients

Indications for conservative treatment:

- Minimally displaced fracture (Not more than 30°),
- Pediatric fractures,
- Presence of systemic comorbidities which may be an absolute contraindication for surgery,
- Condylar head fracture where there is an increased risk of injury to the joint and the adjoining structures. (Vascularity of the fragment may also be compromised by osteosynthesis).
- Minimal pain complaints and no occlusal discrepancies with acceptable range of movements.
- Diacapitular fracture of the condyle [9].

Conservative treatment consists of maxillo-mandibular fixation by means of arch bars, IMF screws or dental splints (cap splint or gunning splint) and inter-maxillary traction using elastics or wires. Immobilization of the joints are done for a period of 4–6 weeks in case of adults whereas 7–10 days for children. Antegrade physiotherapy is mandatory until full adhesion of the fractured fragments [9]. The treatment span is shortened in the pediatric population as they have an increased growth potential and prolonged immobilization may lead to ankylosis of the joint [12].

8.1 Advantages and disadvantages of closed treatment

Advantages:

- Noninvasive, simple, easy to master
- Does not require exposure to general anesthesia
- Economical
- Less chance of infection [13]

Disadvantages:

- Immobilization might not be adequate which delays healing. Especially in subcondylar fractures where control over proximal segments is not established, unfavorable muscle pull can cause displacement of fragments.
- Increases patient morbidity
- Not safe in epileptic patients [13]

9. Surgical treatment of condylar fractures

Conservative treatment using maxillo-mandibular fixation does not always provide satisfactory outcomes. Persistent malocclusion may be present where the necessity for open reduction and internal fixation.

Open reduction and internal fixation helps in faster restoration of both form and function unlike conservative treatment. The patient is rehabilitated in a shorter period of time unlike conservative treatment. Some of the indications for open reduction and internal fixation of mandibular condyle fracture includes.

a. Severe displacement of the condyle

b. Mal-united fracture

c. Bilateral condylar fractures with severe displacement or dislocation affecting the occlusion

d. Associated fractures of the mandible

e. Multifragmented fracture of the condylar head

Zide and Kent's criteria for open reduction are as follows.

Closed reduction	Open reduction
1. Undisplaced or displaced condylar or comminuted fracture (in growing children) where form and function can be restored 2. No medical contraindications for MMF 3. Medical and anesthetic contraindications for open reduction	1. Dislocated condyle and where there is mechanical interferences with the mandibular function 2. Loss of anterior-posterior and vertical dimension that cannot be managed by closed reduction (ex-panfacial and in edentulous fracture) 3. Compound fracture 4. Displacement of condyle into middle cranial fossa 5. Patient and surgeon preference for early or immediate mobilization of function

Table 2.
Indications for open and closed reduction of mandibular condyle fracture AAOMS 2017 guidelines [12].

Absolute indications:

- Displacement of condyle into the middle cranial fossa
- Impossibility of restoring occlusion
- Invasion of foreign body
- Lateral extracapsular displacement

Relative indications:

- When intermaxillary fixation is contraindicated for medical reasons
- Bilateral fracture with open bite deformity
- Bilateral fracture with associated comminuted mid face fracture
- Periodontal problems and loss of teeth
- Unilateral condylar fracture with unstable base [14]

According to AAOMS 2017 the indications for closed and open reduction of condylar fractures are tabulated in **Table 2** [15].

10. Surgical approaches to TMJ

A variety of incisions to approach the TMJ have evolved over the years with each one having their own advantages and disadvantages. These incisions have been categorized into [16]

1. Preauricular and its modification (**Figure 10**)
2. Post-auricular and modification (**Figure 10**)

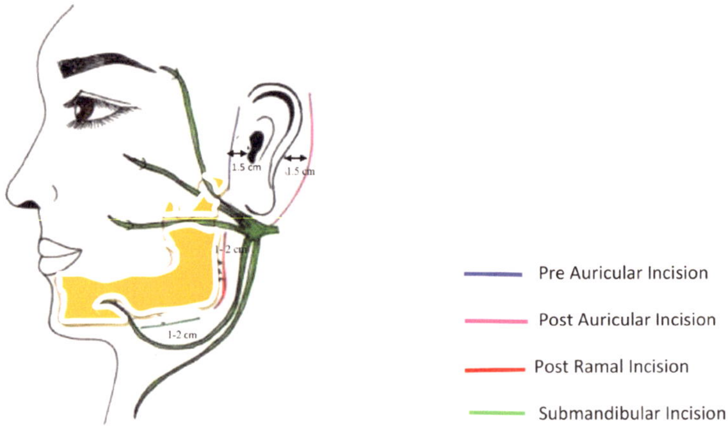

Figure 10.
Approaches to condylar fracture.

3. Endaural and modifications

4. Submandibular (Risdon) (**Figure 10**)

5. Retromandibular or post ramal (**Figure 10**)

6. Rhytidectomy (Face-Lift)

7. Intraoral approach

Approach is based on the level of fracture [17].

The approaches for different levels of fractures with minimal complications are listed below.

- Condylar head fracture—pre-auricular approach or retroauricular approach
- Condylar neck fracture—retromandibular approach with preauricular extension
- Condylar base fracture—submandibular, retromandibular and intra-oral approach

11. Reduction

Reduction is the procedure done for restoring the functional alignment of the fractured bone fragments. Reduction is done to bring the fractured fragments together close to their previous anatomical position so that healing is proper and rapid. Once access is gained to the surgical site reduction is done with the help of bone clamps, forceps, screw and wire and towel clips [13].

12. Fixation

Fixation is the surgical procedure that is done to stabilize and join the ends of fractured bones by mechanical devices such as metal plates, pins, rods, wires, or screws (**Figure 11**).

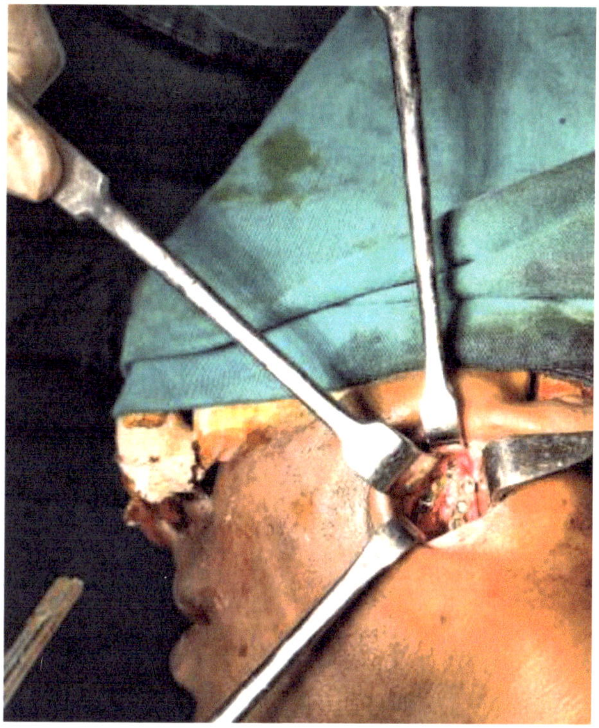

Figure 11.
Miniplate fixation.

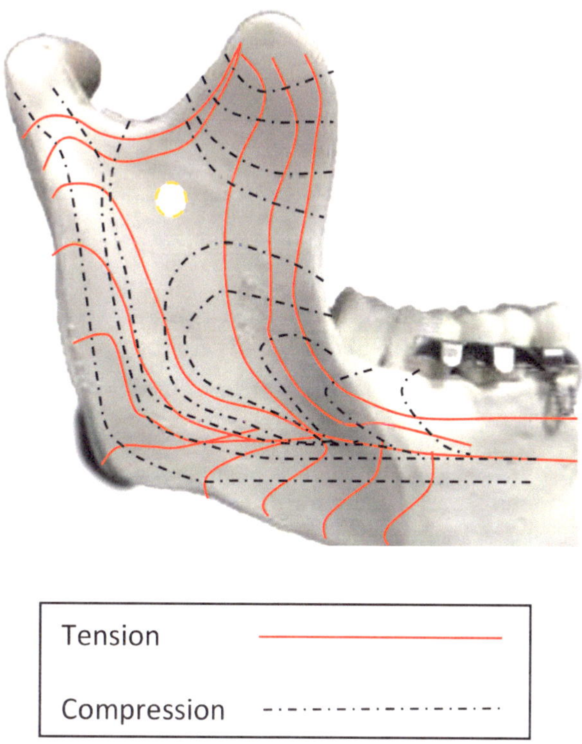

Figure 12.
Zone of tension and compression.

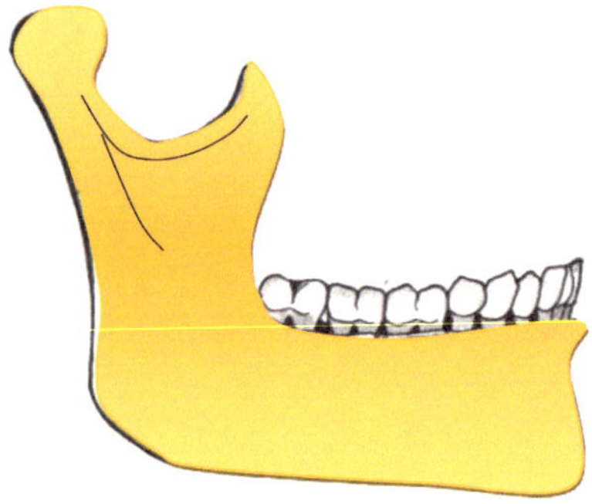

Figure 13.
Ideal line of osteosynthesis.

12.1 Ideal lines of osteosynthesis

The condyles are subjected to major stress during mastication. Meyers gave the ideal lines of osteosynthesis for the mandibular condyle through his research works as follows:

1. Zone of tension: lies along the anterior border of the condyle and the sigmoid notch

2. Zone of compression: lies along the posterior border of the ramus

The long axis of the condylar neck acts as a beam which is subjected to flexion in the sagittal plane. All these biomechanical properties must be taken into consideration while fixation of the fracture pertained to the region (**Figures 12** and **13**) [18].

13. Different fixation options

Fixation is done after ensuring anatomic reduction and normal occlusion.

a. **Single plate—i**n a single miniplate the fracture must be stabilized using two screws on each side of the fracture line. The drawback of this plating has showed the greatest peak displacement of fracture.

b. **Two plates**—application of these two plates at the anterior and posterior aspects of the condylar neck which helps in resisting the torsional force that may not be opposed with a single plate [19].

c. **Geometric plate**—a single L, Y plate, triangular plate, trapezoidal plate, delta plate or 3 D plates are used. Among all plates geometric plates provide the better stability and outcome, because it fulfills the criteria of functionally stable osteosynthesis in the fracture segments [20].

d. **Resorbable plate**—prevents the need for re-operation and has shown good results in the treatment of condylar fractures. They are not very stable when compared to titanium plates in the treatment of condylar fractures [19].

e. **Lag screw**—good clinical results can be obtained especially in diacapitular/sagittal head fractures [21].

f. **Extra corporeal reduction and fixation**—the condyle is explanted from the glenotemporal fossa, reduced and fixed in desired position. The drawback of

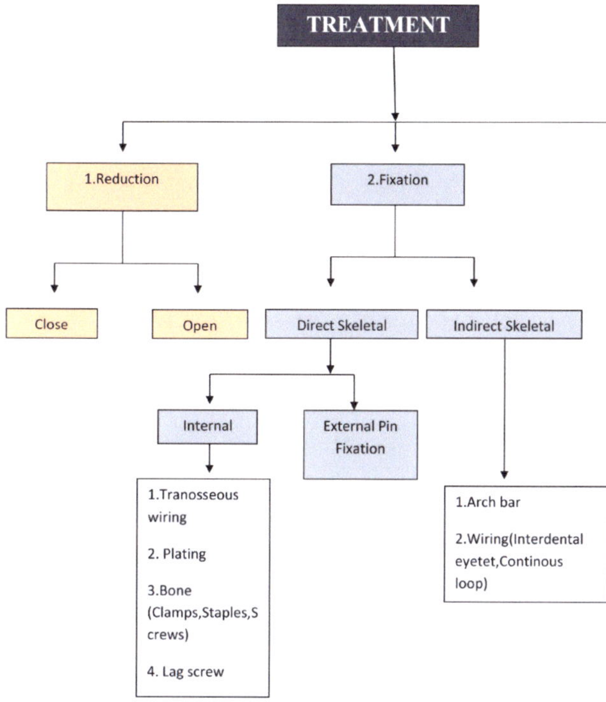

Figure 14.
Treatment algorithm for adult condylar fracture.

this type of fixation will lead to avascular necrosis related to detachment of soft tissue [22].

The treatment plan is summarized and depicted in a flow chart (**Figure 14**) [13].

14. Pediatric condylar fractures

In children displacement of the fractured condyle is uncommon and it is mostly a greenstick fracture. This is due to the fact that the facial bone in children is enclosed by thick soft tissues; the bone is elastic in nature, presence of a large amount of immature trabecular bone and thin cortical bone. Fractures in the pediatric population can easily be overlooked and if untreated may lead to delayed complications like:

1. Ankylosis

2. Poor development of the body and ramus of the mandible on the affected side

3. Gross facial asymmetry

4. Bird face and microgenia in case of bilateral condylar fractures [12]

Treatment in children differs from adults taking the growth and development into consideration. There are certain conditions where surgical treatment is mandatory. Surgical treatment is indicated under the following conditions:

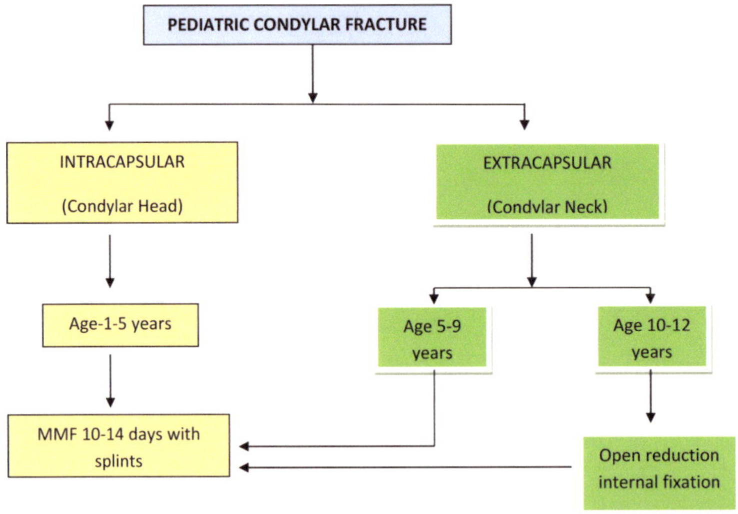

Figure 15.
Treatment algorithm for pediatric condylar fracture.

1. Complex or open fractures

2. Severe displacement

3. Sub condylar fractures with associated facial or calvarial fractures

4. Multiple fractures of the condyle

Surgical treatment may affect the normal growth of the mandible due to the surgical trauma to the soft tissue and the rigidly fixed bony fragments. Moreover, due to the risk of damage to the facial nerve and the invasiveness of surgery conservative treatment is mostly preferred. Maxillomandibular fixation is preferred for a period of 7–10 days followed by physiotherapy (**Figure 15**) [23].

15. Management of geriatric condylar fracture

The cross-sectional area of an atrophic mandible is usually decreased when compared to a mandible with dentition. The vascularity of the bone is decreased and the bone is sclerotic in nature which will hinder or delay the normal healing of the mandible following open reduction. Due to the lack of dentition the fractured fragments are easily displaced. The poor quality of the bone is not suitable for plating the fracture. Conservative treatment with a Gunning splint is advantageous as it provides a stable maxillomandibular fixation and also preserves the periosteal vascularity. Thomas brain gunning designed the "Gunning splint" for maxillomandibular fixation of edentulous or partially edentulous jaw. It consists of two dentures held together in a mono-block. It holds the fracture fragments together and immobilizes the jaw. There is no means of retention or stabilization in an edentulous patient therefore the maxillary denture is secured to the maxilla through per alveolar wiring and the mandibular denture is secured to the mandible with circum-mandibular wiring. The two splints are connected with wire loops or elastics and intermaxillary fixation is achieved [24].

16. Rehabilitation

Rehabilitation can be begun just on the first day of operation in patients who are treated surgically. It mainly consists of exercises which adduces and dissuades the mandible. The exercise is done in front of the mirror so that the mandible is adduced in the correct position. The exercise is done for about 3 to 5 times a day for a timing of 5–10 minutes. In patients who are treated nonsurgically rehabilitation starts at the end of removal of maxillomandibular fixation. Majority of the authors recommend shortening the period of immobilization for 1o to 14 days to prevent the risk of ankylosis. Zaccharides recommends removal of the maxillomandibular fixation once a week during the treatment, the patient should practice opening and closing for half an hour to 1 hour before re-installation of MMF [12]. After conservative treatment physiotherapy is recommended for 3–4 weeks. Rehabilitation is finished when the patient is able to open and close the mouth similar to pre-trauma [9].

17. Complications

Complications in the management of mandibular condyle fractures depends on the severeness of trauma, fracture type, degree of fracture displacement, presence of associated fractures, the type of management (open/closed) and the timing of intervention.

a. Common complications [12]

- Joint motility disorders
- Occlusal discrepancies
- Ipsilateral asymmetry on the side of trauma
- Ankylosis (0.2–0.4%)

b. Rare complications

- Articular head necrosis which is related with surgical method

c. Surgical complications

- Transient or permanent facial palsy
- Marginal mandibular nerve palsy
- Ear lobe hypoesthesia
- Post-surgical scarring
- EAC stenosis
- Formation of sialocele and salivary fistulas
- Auriculotemporal nerve syndrome or Frey's syndrome
- Masseter myotonia

- Mini plate fracture
- Condylar head resorption

The surgical complications are temporary and may persist for about 12 months from the time of operation. Adjunctive pharmacotherapy can be prescribed during this phase (Vitamin B and Vitamin B12 preparations) [9].

18. Conclusion

An appropriate treatment, that is, either a conservative treatment or an open reduction and internal fixation must be considered weighing the advantages and disadvantages, respectively. The treatment must also be based on various factors involved such as age, systemic status, affordability, type of fracture, etc. When a surgical treatment is planned, soft tissue (articular disc) repair must also be considered rather treating the bony component alone as it may lead to delayed temporomandibular joint disorders.

Acknowledgements

We would like to thank Dr. Krishna Kumar Raja, M.D.S. Professor and Head of the Department of Oral and Maxillofacial Surgery, SRM Dental College, for providing us this opportunity.

We would also like to thank Dr. Elavenil Panneerselvam, M.D.S., Reader, Department of Oral and Maxillofacial Surgery, SRM Dental College, for encouraging and guiding us through the entire process.

We would also like to thank Dr. Z.H. Husna Sofia, B.D.S, for providing technical support in the form of diagrams and flowcharts.

Conflict of interest

The authors declare no conflict of interest.

Author details

Kasi Ganesh Sriraam* and K. Rajendran Arun Vignesh
Department of Oral and Maxillofacial Surgery, SRM Dental College and Hospital, Chennai, India

*Address all correspondence to: sriraamkg@gmail.com

References

[1] Sawazaki R, Júnior SM, Asprino L, Moreira RW, De Moraes M. Incidence and patterns of mandibular condyle fractures. Journal of Oral and Maxillofacial Surgery. 2010;**68**(6):1252-1259

[2] Nørholt SE, Krishnan V, Sindet-Pedersen S, Jensen IB. Pediatric condylar fractures: A long-term follow-up study of 55 patients. Journal of Oral and Maxillofacial Surgery. 1993;**51**(12):1302-1310

[3] Barde D, Mudhol A, Madan R. Prevalence and pattern of mandibular fracture in Central India. National Journal of Maxillofacial Surgery. 2014;**5**(2):153

[4] Rozylo-Kalinowska I, Orhan K. Imaging of the Temporomandibular Joint. Switzerland: Springer Nature Switzerland AG; 2019

[5] Hupp J, Tucker M, Ellis E. Contemporary Oral and Maxillofacial Surgery. Philadelphia: Elsevier; 2019

[6] Powers DB. Classification of mandibular condylar fractures. Atlas of the Oral and Maxillofacial Surgery Clinics of North America. 2017;**25**(1):1-10

[7] Neff A, Cornelius CP, Rasse M, Torre D, Audigé L. The comprehensive AOCMF classification system: Condylar process fractures-level 3 tutorial. Craniomaxillofacial Trauma & Reconstruction. 2014;**7**(S01):S044-S058

[8] Ying BB, Zhang QQ, Zhu SS, Li YF. Outcomes of treatment for intracapsular fractures of the mandibular condyle: Recommendation for a new classification. The British Journal of Oral & Maxillofacial Surgery. 2018;**56**(2):139-143

[9] Niedzielska I, Tomczyk-Wziątek A, Borowski B. Fractures of the mandibular condylar processes—Literature review. Open Medicine. 2013;**8**(2):244-249

[10] Naeem A, Gemal H, Reed D. Imaging in traumatic mandibular fractures. Quantitative Imaging in Medicine and Surgery. 2017;**7**(4):469

[11] Ren R, Dai J, Si J, Cai B, Shi J. Changes of disc status in adult patients with condylar head fracture who did or did not undergo disc anchoring operation. Journal of Cranio-Maxillofacial Surgery. 2018;**46**(12):2248-2255

[12] Zachariades N, Mezitis M, Mourouzis C, Papadakis D, Spanou A. Fractures of the mandibular condyle: A review of 466 cases. Literature review, reflections on treatment and proposals. Journal of Cranio-Maxillofacial Surgery. 2006;**34**(7):421-432

[13] Banks P, Killey H. Killey's Fractures of the Mandible. Oxford, England: Wright; 1991

[14] Brandt MT, Haug RH. Open versus closed reduction of adult mandibular condyle fractures: A review of the literature regarding the evolution of current thoughts on management. Journal of Oral and Maxillofacial Surgery. 2003;**61**(11):1324-1332

[15] Ochs M, Chung W, Powers D. Trauma surgery. Journal of Oral and Maxillofacial Surgery. 2017;**75**(8):e151-e194

[16] Quinn P, Granquist E. Atlas of Temporomandibular Joint Surgery. 2nd ed. New Jersey, United states: John Wiley & Sons; 2015

[17] Al-Moraissi EA, Louvrier A, Colletti G, et al. Does the surgical approach for treating mandibular condylar fractures affect the rate of seventh cranial nerve injuries? A

systematic review and meta-analysis based on a new classification for surgical approaches. Journal of Cranio-Maxillo-Facial Surgery. 2018;**46**(3):398-412

[18] Meyer C, Martin E, Jean-Luc KA, Simone ZI. Development and biomechanical testing of a new osteosynthesis plate (TCP®) designed to stabilize mandibular condyle fractures. Journal of Cranio-Maxillofacial Surgery. 2007;**35**(2):84-90

[19] Bischoff EL, Carmichael R, Reddy LV. Plating options for fixation of condylar neck and base fractures. Atlas of the Oral and Maxillofacial Surgery Clinics of North America. 2017;**25**(1):69-73

[20] Bhowmick RS, Bhowal K, Ghosh S. Plating systems for 3D stability of subcondylar fracture: A research article with review of literature. International Journal of Orthopaedics. 2019;**5**(2):681-683

[21] Kallela I, Söderholm AL, Paukku P, Lindqvist C. Lag-screw osteosynthesis of mandibular condyle fractures: A clinical and radiological study. Journal of Oral and Maxillofacial Surgery. 1995;**53**(12):1397-1404

[22] Park JM, Jang YW, Kim SG, et al. Comparative study of the prognosis of an extracorporeal reduction and a closed treatment in mandibular condyle head and/or neck fractures. Journal of Oral and Maxillofacial Surgery. 2010;**68**(12):2986-2993

[23] Choi KY, Yang JD, Chung HY, Cho BC. Current concepts in the mandibular condyle fracture management part II: Open reduction versus closed reduction. Archives of Plastic Surgery. 2012;**39**(4):301

[24] Sharma B, Sharma P, Goswami R, Jain S, Samra RK. Construction of a gunning splint; case report on the handling of mandibular fractures in edentulous patients. Indian Journal of Dental Sciences. 2020;**12**:36-39

Chapter 8

Alveolar Ridge Augmentation Techniques in Implant Dentistry

Melike Aytekin and Volkan Arisan

Abstract

Implant supported restorations have become an ideal treatment alternative for the rehabilitation of edentulous sites. However alveolar bone defects due to resorption, trauma or oncologic diseases may considerably affect favorable implant positioning and prosthetic outcomes. Various alveolar ridge augmentation procedures are available to gain enough bone volume and apply the ideal treatment plan afterwards. Guided bone regeneration, ridge splitting, distraction osteogenesis, maxillary sinus augmentation and autogenous block bone grafting are main techniques which have successful outcomes in reconstruction of bone defects. It's difficult to demonstrate that one augmentation procedure offers better outcomes than another. Studies documenting augmentation techniques seem to be comparable and state favorable results for each procedure.

Keywords: biomaterials, alveolar ridge deficiency, distraction osteogenesis, ridge splitting, guided bone regeneration, onlay block bone graft

1. Introduction

Dental implant supported prosthetic rehabilitation has become a widely used treatment option in partial and completely edentulous patients as recent advances occur in materials and techniques. Hard and soft tissue defects are usually present in these edentulous patients due to a variety of traumatic events such as periodontal diseases, oncologic pathologies and tooth loss. Ridge augmentation procedures may be necessary before or during the implant surgery to overcome the challenges arising from bony defects and achieve ideal implant positioning with predictable treatment outcomes (**Figure 1**).

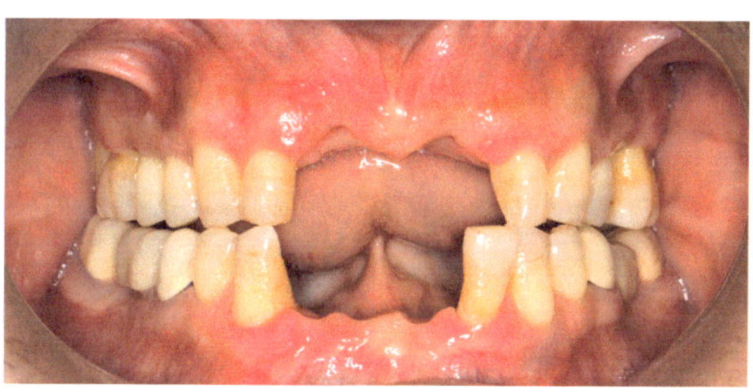

Figure 1.
Loss of anterior teeth resulting with severe loss of alveolar bone. Bone volume should be restored for the proper restoration of the lost teeth.

A large variety of bone augmentation techniques can be applied in the presence of bone defects. Guided bone regeneration, ridge splitting, distraction osteogenesis, maxillary sinus lifting and autogenous onlay block bone grafting are main techniques which have successful outcomes in reconstruction of bone defects. This chapter reviews alveolar ridge augmentation techniques in brief [1–4].

Defect morphology plays a critical role when choosing the type of augmentation procedure to perform. Number of surrounding bony walls are important when an augmentation is planned, because vascularization and healing properties are provided by these walls to the augmentation site. Therefore, defects with less amount of remaining bony walls are considered to be complex [5, 6].

1.1 Classification of defect morphology

Classification of the defect morphology is as follows [5]:

- *Thick five bony wall defect* is usually a tooth extraction socket. This type of defects have most of the important keys for a predictable bone regeneration process. Defect size is small, therefore regeneration by particulate bone grafts is possible. Surrounding five bony walls provide space maintenance and stabilize the blood clot along with the graft particulates. Torn blood vessels post-extraction accelerates the regeneration by releasing growth factors to the site. Augmentation of five bony wall defect is preservation of the residual alveolar ridge. Any resorbable graft material can be used in this type of bone defect depending on the desired healing period until the implant placement.

- Regeneration of *four to five bony wall defect* is impaired since vascularization from bony walls is reduced and partially replaced by soft tissue vascularization. When the buccal wall is missing post-extraction, space maintenance is no longer possible by the socket itself. Soft tissue tends to grow into the socket, therefore use of a barrier membrane along with particulate bone grafts is necessary to regain the ideal volume and contour of bone. Any resorbable bone graft material can be preferred in this case. When one of the lateral walls is missing following extraction, repair of this wall can be faciliated with socket preservation procedure at the time of extraction. Otherwise, during the healing period residual bone resorption may occur to an extend that requires further augmentation procedures.

- Treatment of *two to three bony wall defect* is similar to the treatment of four bony wall defect. Since the defect size is bigger in this type, use of autogenous bone grafts is required for their osteogenic properties. It's recommended to combine autografts with other resorbable graft materials to avoid rapid resorption and provide enough space while new bone regenerates. Resorbable barrier membranes can be supported with tenting screws or titanium reinforced non-resorbable membranes can be preferred in this type of defects as it requires more stability and space maintenance for longer periods.

- *One bony wall defect* is the most challenging defect type. Vascularization and regeneration potential of this defect is very low. Bone volume that needs to be regenerated is at high levels. For predictable outcomes, it's recommended to fixate onlay bone blocks to the host bone in this type of severe bone atrophies. There are studies reporting better outcomes with utilizing both onlay bone block grafting and guided bone regeneration at the same time [7] (**Figure 2**).

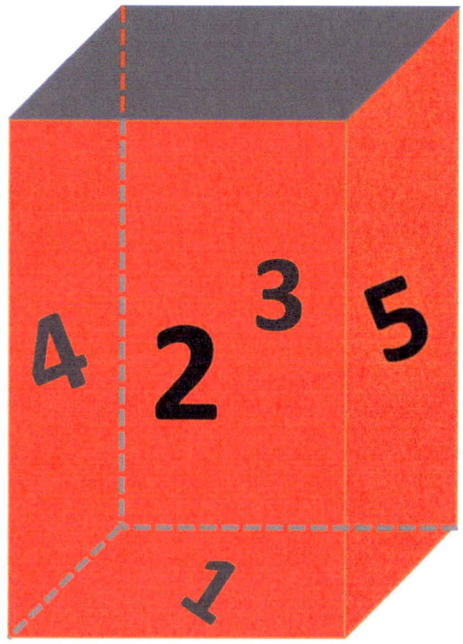

Figure 2.
Schematic representation of a five-walled bone defect. A reduce in the number of any walls renders corresponding wall-numbered bone defect. Translation of this wall-wall-number defect classification to the clinical scenario may not always be straight-forward.

2. Guided bone regeneration

Guided bone regeneration (GBR) is a procedure utilizing barrier membranes to create adequate space for new bone formation. Use of barrier membranes avoids soft tissue collapse and non-osteogenic cell migration into the bone defect [8]. It also facilitates an ideal environment for bone formation by providing space maintenance, stabilization of graft materials and prevention of soft tissue ingrowth (**Figure 3**) [9]. Guided bone regeneration can is indicated for the augmentation of [8]:

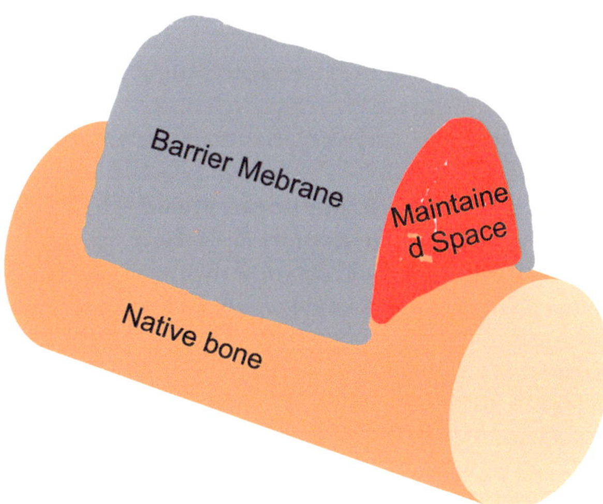

Figure 3.
Guided bone regeneration (GBR) procedure create and maintain a space via a semi-permiable barrier membrane which the blood cloth will occupy and allow the proliferation of the bone-producing cells.

- Vertical bone defects
- Horizontal bone defects
- Fenestration bone defects
- Dehiscence bone defects
- Combined vertical and horizontal defects
- Circumferential peri-implantitis defects
- Extraction sites

Over a decade, autogenous bone block grafting was the standard procedure in augmentation of bone defects. Due to its' invasive harvesting technique, morbidity at the donor site and limited availability, new techniques are developed. With rapid progress in biomaterials, GBR became one of the safest and most common techniques as it's less invasive and causes less discomfort post-operatively. Particulate grafts used in the procedure can easily be adapted into complex defect geometries [2, 5]. Urban et al. demonstrated a new bone formation of 5.45 mm vertically as a mean value when GBR protocol is performed utilizing xenograft and autogenous particulate graft mix with d-PTFE membranes [10]. Still, GBR has its own technique-sensitive challenges and is need to be practiced meticulously.

To achieve successful and repetitive outcomes, guided bone regeneration has 4 key principles: P-A-S-S [2, 8].

Primary wound closure is an important key factor for an optimal healing and success. In the augmentation sites, biomaterials and membranes increase the tissue volume so it becomes harder to close the wound without tension.

To provide a tension-free closure, incision design must be considered carefully.

- Incision should be kept within the keratinized tissue as much as possible.
- Vertical releasing incisions should be as far as possible from the augmentation site and help create a wide-base flap.
- Subperiosteal scoring incision and flap release should be performed.

Angiogenesis provide nutrients and oxygen to the augmentation site and enhances healing process in this way. To ensure an ideal angiogenesis, patients must be examined thoroughly in terms of systemic diseases which affect healing mechanisms such as diabetes mellitus and osteoporosis. In these cases, an internist or an endocrinologist may be consulted if necessary. Any uncontrolled systemic disease should be taken into consideration as a contraindication. Smoking habits also reduce vascularization and proper blood supply in the surgical site. Measures like using local anesthetics without vasoconstrictors or encouraging patients to regulate their smoking cycles can be taken.

Space creation and maintenance prevents soft tissue collapse to the surgical site thus osteogenic cells can proliferate and gradually form bone tissue. Biomaterials and particulate grafts along with barrier membranes can be used for this process. While barrier membranes prevent migration of soft tissue cells to the regeneration space, bone grafts and biomaterials provide structural strength. Depending on the type of barrier membrane in use, tenting poles can be used to provide additional strength.

Stability of wound clot is essential for optimal healing since the blood clot provides lots of growth factors to the surgical site. Primary wound closure and barrier membranes, acting as a roof to the regeneration site, contribute in stabilizing the blood clot. Recent studies show that barrier membranes need to be fixated with pins or screws to provide enough stability also to the graft materials, otherwise up to %40 of graft content is lost until the patient leaves the clinic [11, 12].

2.1 Barrier membranes

A barrier membrane is an essential component in guided bone regeneration procedures. Various membranes with different features are available on the market [12]. Barrier membranes should fulfill some basic requirements to be safely utilized in dental applications [3].

- *Biocompability:* Host tissue and membrane should be biologically compatible avoiding any foreign body reactions.
- *Space-maintenance:* Barrier membrane must avoid any collapse and maintain space during the regeneration period.
- *Barrier function:* Preventing soft tissue cells from migrating to regeneration site is an essential feature for membranes.
- *Stability:* Membranes must have mechanical strength and proper physical properties which protects the regeneration site during healing period.
- *Degradability:* Ideally a membrane should degrade at a time rate matching the regeneration period.

There are two main groups of membranes: resorbable and non-resorbable [7].

2.1.1 Resorbable membranes

Using resorbable membranes eliminates the second surgical intervention for membrane removal after healing and in this way decreases morbidity. Less complications occur with resorbable membranes compared to the non-resorbable ones. These membranes can easily be manipulated and adapted to the defect since they don't have any reinforcements with high elastic modulus. On the other hand, when compared to non-resorbable membranes they are more prone to collapse which lowers the maintained space. Bone graft substitutes and additional tools like tenting poles can be used along with resorbable membranes to increase stability. One major drawback of these membranes is varied and sometimes unpredictable resorption rates which directly affect new bone formation [13–15].

Resorbable membranes can be classified as natural and synthetic (**Figure 4**).

- *Non-cross-linking resorbable collagen membranes* are made of native collagen, have high levels of biocompability. They well-integrate into tissues and rapidly become vascularized. However, non-cross-linking resorbable membranes may resorp earlier than the required time for regeneration and lose their barrier functions. Cellular activity of host bone, membrane properties and possible exposures affect the biodegradation time. If any exposure occurs within the membrane, soft tissue spontaneously covers the exposed area in most cases. Bone grafts may resorp causing a decrease in the expected bone formation, though [3, 13].

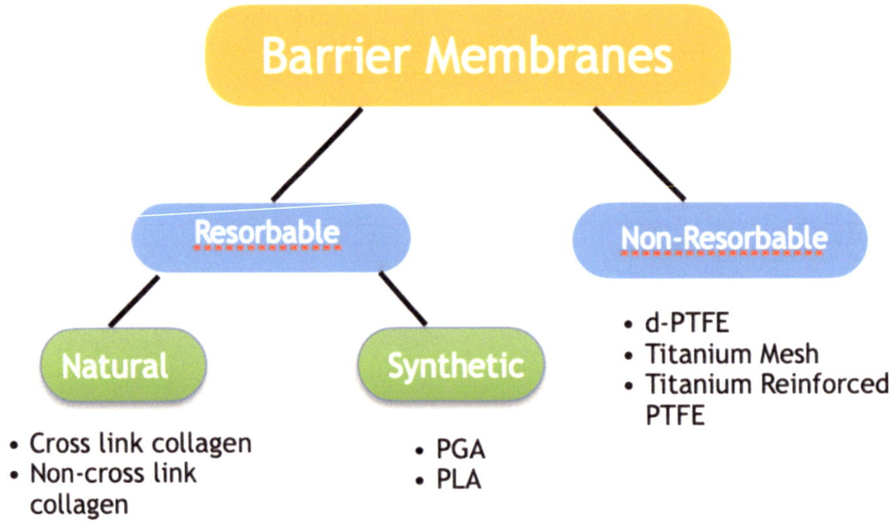

Figure 4.
Classification of barrier membranes used in guided bone regeneration procedures.

- *Cross-linked resorbable collagen membranes* are rich in cross-linking collagen fibrils so their degradation time is extended. Increased amount of collagen fibrils result in less biocompatibility and harder manipulation, still studies state good results in tissue integration and bone regeneration using these membranes [13–16].

- *Synthetic resorbable membranes*, mainly consisting of polyesters like polylactic acid or polyglycolic acid copolymers, are produced to achieve extended biodegradation period and increased biocompability. Derived from various origins, these membranes can offer various physical, chemical and mechanical properties. They also differ from natural resorbable membranes in terms of degradation pathways. Tatakis et al. demonstrated that synthetic resorbable membranes degrade via hydrolisis and alteration of degradation products through citric acid cycle causes an acidic enviroment. Therefore, using synthetic resorbable membranes result in higher inflammatory response and complications of soft tissue perforation [3, 13].

2.1.2 Non-resorbable membranes

When a bone defect lacks several supportive adjacent walls, utilized barrier membrane should provide additional strength to maintain space and stay stable during the regeneration process. To ensure stability and structural strength, different materials and compositions are used in production of non-resorbable membranes: titanium mesh, e-PTFE, d-PTFE and titanium reinforced PTFE membranes [3].

- **Expanded polytetrafluoroethylene (e-PTFE)** is the first generation of non-resorbable membranes used for guided bone regeneration. It's mostly preferred when a critical size defect is present and high amount of grafting is needed. Their stiff form makes them less compatible with soft tissues causing high rates of exposure. Once an exposure occurs with these membranes in use, infection develops and due to the porous structure, mechanical or chemical cleaning of infected site is almost impossible whether at early or late stage of healing. Recently, these membranes are rarely used in oral surgical interventions due to the high infection and irreversible complication rates [5, 7, 13].

- **Dense polytetrafluoroethylene (d-PTFE) membranes** are produced to overcome the disadvantages of e-PTFE membranes. These membranes have smaller pore size that they don't allow microorganism migration while oxygen diffusion is still possible in case of an exposure. With their low infection rates and additional mechanical strength, these micro-porous non-resorbable membranes are found to be effective in guided bone regeneration procedures [3, 13, 17]. Ronda et al. reported a mean defect fill of 5.49 mm in vertically augmented sites using d-PTFE membranes 6 months post-operatively [18].

- **Titanium mesh membranes** are porous titanium plates used in guided bone regeneration. The pores in these membranes are large and do not interfere with blood supply. Ti mesh is highly biocompatible to the surrounding tissues. Infection rates are very low with these membranes. They have a wide range of properties like rigidity, elasticity, stability and plasticity which exceptionally make these membranes adaptable but rigid at the same time. Titanium mesh membranes are commonly used in large bone defects and when a resistance to the pressure of soft tissue is needed to avoid collapse. Main disadvantage of Ti mesh membranes is high exposure rates due to their stiffness, several studies reported different exposure rates up to %50 [3, 17, 19].

- **Titanium reinforced PTFE membranes** are modifications of PTFE membranes. There are titanium frameworks embedded in these membranes for additional strength and rigidity therefore they successfully maintain space during the healing period and do not collapse. They are mostly used for vertical bone augmentation where additional resistance to soft tissue collapse is crucial. Added framework results in higher rates of exposure [3, 20].

2.2 Bone grafting materials

Various bone grafts and biomaterials can be used in guided bone regeneration. To choose the right material for predictable results in augmentation procedures, how these materials induce bone healing should be well-known. Healing properties of bone grafts and biomaterials are classified into three categories: osteogenesis, osteoinduction, osteoconduction [3, 5, 8].

2.2.1 Osteogenesis

Osteogenesis is defined as formation of new bone through viable osteoblast cells transferred to the site within grafting material. Autogenous bone grafts are transplanted from one site to another and the only type of grafting material with osteogenic features. Compared to cortical bone grafts, cancellous bone grafts contain higher amounts of osteoblast cells. To maintain the vitality of these cells and the dependent osteogenic process, angiogenesis is critically important. Therefore, once the autogenous bone graft is harvested it should be stored in sterile saline solution and placed in the recipient site as soon as possible. There are studies stating that autogenous bone grafts lose their osteogenic properties in 5 days without vascular support [5, 13].

2.2.2 Osteoinduction

Osteoinduction is a process where grafting material induces mesenchymal stem cells to migrate, proliferate and differentiate into osteoprogenitor cells. With osteoprogenitor cells occuring in the site, new bone forms [5, 13].

Urist et al. performed the landmark study on osteoinductive grafting materials isolating bone morphogenetic protein (BMP), a growth factor from the transforming growth factor (TGF)-β family, and described it as the main inductive agent [5, 21, 22].

2.2.3 Osteoconduction

Osteoconduction refers to bone growth into a scaffold formed by the grafting material [5]. It's characterized by resorption of the grafting material and apposition of the new bone which is called "creeping substitution" process. Osteoconductive graft materials are biocompatible and contains osteoconductive surfaces such as pores, tubes and ducts so that the surronding bone can grow into these spaces. This type of grafting materials have no potential of bone growth by itself but take part in the regeneration process as a supporting structure [3, 5, 22, 23].

2.2.4 Types of grafting materials

Various types of grafting materials are available for use in bone augmentation procedures (**Figure 5**). With different action mechanisms and regeneration potentials, there is no definitive recommendation specific to any procedure. Results vary depending on the regenerative approaches in conjunction with grafting materials. The most common classification for bone graft materials is as follows [3]:

- Autografts (same individual)

- Allografts (human cadaver source)

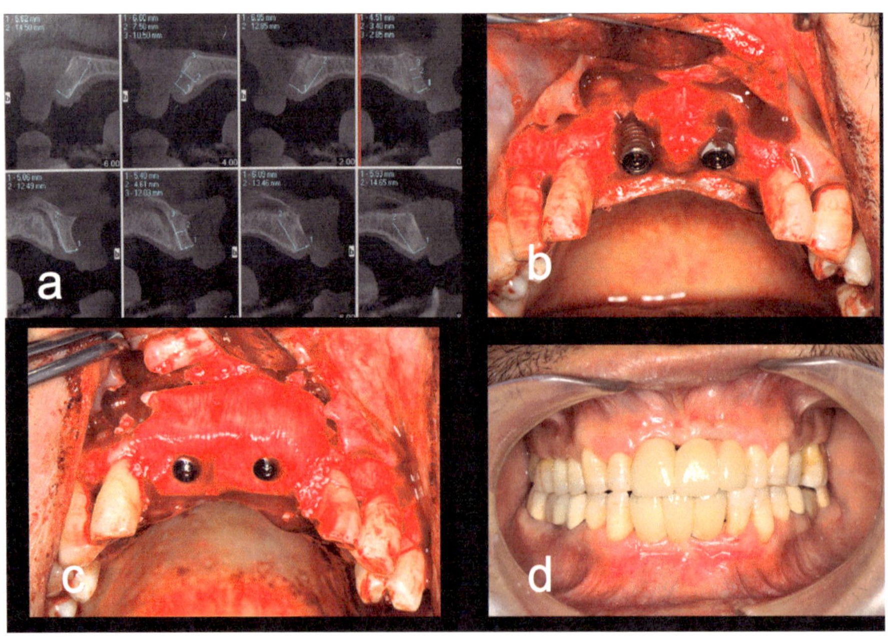

Figure 5.
Restoration of missing maxillary incisors (clinical view in **Figure 1***) via GBR and titanium dental implants. (a) tomogram reveal severe bone atrophy, (b) dental implants showing insufficient bone coverage, (c) GBR procedure covering the area of missing bone volume stabilized on to the dental implants, (d) final prosthetic restoration.*

- Xenografts (animal source)
- Alloplasts (synthetic source)

2.2.4.1 Autografts

Autogenous grafts, also known as autografts, are type of grafts transferred from one site to another within the same individual. These grafts are harvested in the form of bone blocks or particulates. Main intraoral donor sites are mandibular symphisis, ramus buccal shelf and maxillar tuberosity. They can either be harvested from iliac crest, calvaria, tibial plates and costae extraorally when larger volumes of autograft is required [2, 3].

Containing viable osteoblast cells, these materials are the only grafting materials with osteogenic properties. Therefore they have capacity of bone growth in the recipient site when vascularized. During incorporation growth factors, such as bone morphogenetic proteins, are released and induce bone growth through osteoinduction mechanism. Subsequently, a part of autograft becomes nonviable and acts as a scaffold with its calcium phosphate matrix. Surrounding bone is conducted by this matrix to regenerate. So autografts acts in all three mechanisms: osteogenesis, osteoinduction and osteoconduction [2, 24].

Main advantages of autografts are low cost, unique osteogenic properties and early vascularization. Although autografts are considered to be a golden standard for augmentation procedures, search and evaluation for new grafting materials continue due to secondary surgical site for harvesting, limited source, morbidity and infection risk at the donor site. In contrast, a number of comparative studies reported autografts to remain golden standard for augmentation procedures due to their rapid stimulation of new bone formation compared to other bone grafting materials [3, 5, 13].

2.2.4.2 Allografts

Allografts are transferred from an individual to another within the same species. Since there is no need for a secondary surgical site to obtain allografts, reduced morbidity is one of the advantages brought by use of this graft. Unlimited source is another advantage over autografts. Although allografts have no osteogenic properties, they stimulate bone growth via osteoconduction and incorporation of osteoinductive growth factors. There are strict sterilization and decontamination protocols regarding these materials due to the risk of disease transmission and host immune response. Donors are carefully evaluated and graft materials are gradually processed to avoid any risks. Some studies reported that certain allografts are less osteoinductive than others because of the sterilization protocols and the variability of their content. Schwartz et al. studied on different allografts taken from various tissue banks and stated wide range of variability related to donor's age, preparation method and sterilization protocols [2, 3].

There are four forms of allografts: fresh frozen bone, freeze-dried bone allograft, demineralized free-dried bone allograft and deproteinized bone allograft.

Freeze-dried bone allografts (FDBA) and demineralized freeze-dried bone allografts (DFDBA) are more frequently in use. DFDBA is demineralized with hydrochloric acid to provide easier access to growth factors such as BMP thus increase osteoinductive potential. Due to the lack of mineralized content, disadvantage of rapid resorption arises with DFDBA use. For this reason, FDBA is utilized more routinely in bone augmentation procedures. Compared to DFDBA, it's easier to track FDBA on radiographs with it's mineralized and radiopaque characteristics. Therefore, it's easier document this material's follow-up and resorption rates [5, 24].

2.2.4.3 Xenografts

Grafts obtained from different species like bovine animals are called xenografts. This type of grafts are deproteinized to avoid the risk of disease transmission and they are present in spongeous form. Deproteinized bovine bone mineral (DBBM) is the most utilized and well-documented type of xenograft. Since it's highly purified, anorganic and protein-free, it has no osteogenic potential nor osteoinductive properties. DBBM contains natural calcium phosphate which facilitates osteoconduction. Mineral content of this graft material provides low rates of resorption over time. Due to their long-term low resorption features, there is a widespread use of xenografts in augmentation procedures where the healing period is long and space maintenance is needed during this time. Sinus augmentations, contour augmentations, augmentation of horizontal and vertical defects are among the procedures xenografts can be preferred. Several studies demonstrated that DBBM particulates are present in the regeneration site up to 10 years after the placement [7, 13, 25]. In a study conducted by Mendoza-Azpur et al., GBR cases utilizing xenografts alone and along with autogenous block bones are evaluated. Results demonstrated statistically no significant difference between two groups in terms of implant survival rates. Higher rate of complications and post-operative discomfort is reported in the group receiving autogenous block bones, though [26].

2.2.4.4 Alloplasts

Alloplastic biomaterials are produced in the laboratories synthetically to avoid the disadvantages of allografts and xenografts. Providing space maintenance and acting as a scaffold, they stimulate osteoconduction. Biocompatibility, zero risk for disease transmission and availability are important advantages of these biomaterials. There are resorbable and non-resorbable forms of alloplasts. For resorbable alloplasts, porosity of the material is the main factor that affects resorption rate; increased micro-porosity leads to faster turnover. Although non-resorbable alloplasts are seldomly used alone as the grafting material in augmentation procedures, resorbable alloplasts show good results used either alone or in combination with other grafting materials since they act as a scaffold and provide stability to the regeneration site. These materials are derived from the combinations of hydroxyapatite (HA), β-TCP, polymers and/or bioactive glasses [5, 24].

Synthetic hydroxyapatites are biomaterials similar to the human bone in terms of chemical composition. Therefore they cause minimal inflammation and foreign body reactions. With their high levels of chemical stability and biocompatibility, they can be used in many clinical applications such as ridge preservation following extraction or ridge augmentation to reconstruct bone defects. One of the important advantages of this material is the possibility of altering the microstructure and new bone formation accordingly [3, 5, 13].

Calcium phosphate ceramics are promising biomaterials considering their high level of biocompatibility, low risk of foreign body reactions and possibility of combination with bioactive molecules and therapeutic agents. Hydroxyapatite layer forms after the placement of calcium phosphate ceramics faciliating osteoinduction in addition to osteoconduction mechanism. Although alloplastic materials have many advantages, these materials demonstrate lower regenerative potential in comparison with other grafting materials [3]. Further studies are required to document these biomaterials [3, 27].

2.3 Growth factors

Bone augmentation procedures are advanced and complex surgical interventions. Since there are multiple factors affecting the treatment outcomes, growth factors which promote healing and regeneration are mostly used along with the grafting materials and membranes. These agents are widely utilized especially when bone healing mechanisms are affected by the patient's medical conditions such as diabetes mellitus or osteoporosis. Growth factors used in dentistry are divided in two categories: platelet concentrates and recombinant growth factors [3, 5, 28].

2.3.1 Platelet concentrates

Platelet concentrates are obtained by centrifuging autologous blood to concentrate platelets, cells taking part in the active secretion of growth factors. These concentrates have two forms as platelet-rich plasma (PRP) and platelet-rich fibrin (PRF) [3].

PRP is the first generation of platelet concentrates consisting %95 platelets, %4 red blood cells and %1 white blood cells. Although PRP has been widely used for it's healing enhancing properties for a long time, it's observed to have some major drawbacks. Several studies reported that incorporation of bovine thrombin or calcium chloride as anticoagulants decelerates the healing process and poses a risk for infection transmission or host immune response. It's preparation method is demanding and technique-sensitive. Furthermore, there are studies showing rapid release of growth factors from PRP whereas the desired release process is extended and gradual to cover the regenerative phase. PRF is developed to overcome these limitations [28].

PRF is obtained without any anticoagulant use, therefore it's a fibrin matrix containing the full set of growth factors in it's matrix. Fibrin form of this platelet concentrate facilitates a slow release of growth factors over time as desired. PRF, later called as L-PRF, is rich in leukocytes and platelets. High levels of leukocytes contribute in wound healing and vascular formation along with their contribution in host defense to pathogens at the regeneration site as they are anti-infectious and immune modulating cells [29].

L-PRF is easily prepared compared to PRP. Once the blood sample is collected, it's put in glass tubes and centrifuged at 750 g for 12 minutes. It's important to centrifuge the collection quickly, since the sample's contact with glass tube walls starts the coagulation process rapidly. When the centrifugation is complete, there are three layers in the tube: red blood cells in the bottom, cells plasma at the top and L-PRF in the middle [13, 30].

With it's fibrin matrix structure acting as a scaffold for tissue ingrowth, rich content in cells recruiting future regenerative cells to the site and gradual delivery of growth factors make L-PRF attractive for use in regeneration procedures (**Figure 6**) [31, 32].

2.3.2 Recombinant growth factors

Bone morphogenetic protein (BMP) is a well-documented recombinant growth factor with it's recruiting, proliferating and differentiating effect on mesenchymal progenitor cells. Studies show osteoinductive properties of BMP activates osteoblast differentiation pathway MAPK/ERK. It's capacity of osteoinduction is at higher levels compared to other known growth factors therefore BMP can be utilized to promote bone regeneration especially in complex augmentation procedures like vertical augmentation [13, 33].

Platelet-derived growth factor (PDGF) is the second most utilized growth factor in augmentation procedures. It's responsible for cell migration and proliferation to

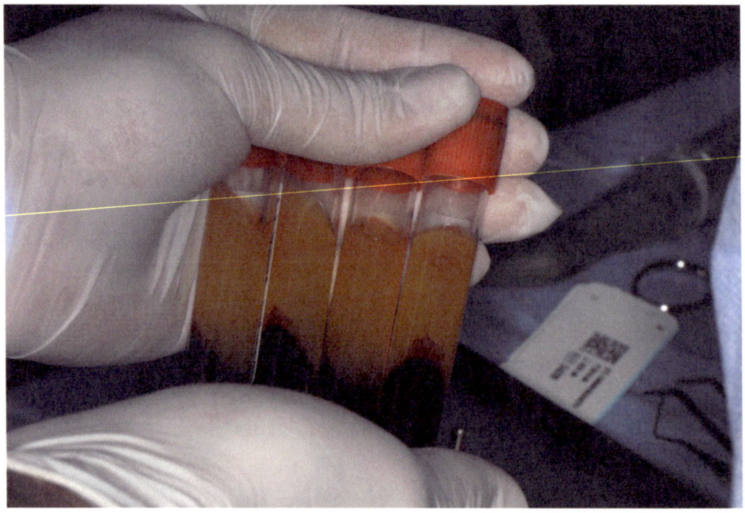

Figure 6.
Prepared human blood-derived PRF in the centrifuge tubes.

the defect site. Several studies reported PDGF to be highly effective on regeneration in advanced periodontal osseous defects [3].

3. Autogenous onlay block bone grafting

In many bone defects, guided bone regeneration procedures result in successful outcomes. It has several superiorities over block bone grafting like eliminating the secondary surgical site for bone harvesting and post-operative discomfort at the donor site. However, GBR is well-documented in regeneration of new bone up to 4.5–5 mm width and height. When the defect size gets larger, it's harder to achieve predictable results with this protocol. Although extending the healing period is recommended in large size defects, new bone quality is still observed to be less than ideal. Also GBR covering full arches, especially mandible, is not predictable. Therefore autogenous block bone grafting is utilized in large size defects [11, 34].

Significant amount (>5 mm) of new bone formation in vertical or horizontal dimensions can be achieved utilizing autogenous bone block grafting. It is indicated in augmentation of severely atrophic crests. In a review by Aloy-Prosper et al., autogenous block bone grafting procedures and their results are evaluated. In horizontally augmented sites utilizing block bones, implant survival rates are found to be ranging from %96.9 and %100. In vertically augmented sites through same procedures, implant survival rates are slightly lower ranging from %89.5 and %100 [35].

Autografts to be used in the procedure are obtained from various donor sites intra- and extraorally. Less complications are reported when intraoral donor sites are preferred for harvesting. When deciding for the donor site, amount of needed bone volume and defect size should be carefully evaluated. Autogenous bone graft shows high resorption rates, therefore it's important to harvest larger volumes considering the possible resorption [5]. Despite high resorption rates, osteogenic potential of autogenous bone makes this procedure feasible. Comparing GBR with autogenous block bone grafting, Jensen et al. reported that reaugmentation is needed in %11.1 of GBR cases and %2.8 of block bone grafting cases due to insufficient new bone formation [36]. Recently, there are studies recommending combination of autogenous block bone grafting and GBR. Chappuis et al. clinically and radiographically evaluated GBR in combination with autogenous block bone grafting. %98.1 success rate and a minimal block graft resorption rate of %7.7 is reported in 10 years post-operatively [37].

3.1 Intraoral donor sites

Mandibular symphisis, buccal ramus shelf, maxillary tuberosity and torus are the main intraoral sources for bone block harvesting. Membranous grafts such as grafts obtained from mandibula are reported to have less resorption rates than the endochondrial grafts obtained from extraoral sites. Dimensional stability of the new bone and incorporation of grafts to the host site is also shown to be better when membranous grafts are utilized. Main advantages of intraoral bone blocks are less occuring complications, no need for patients to go under general anesthesia, no cutaneous scarring, easy surgical access, less morbidity in the donor site and more content of bone growth factors [38–41].

3.1.1 Intraoral harvest from ramus

Block bone grafts harvested from ramus are cortical type. Around 10–15 mm thick and 4 cm long blocks can be harvested from ramus. Maximum thickness of the bone block is defined by the distance between external oblique line and inferior alveolar nerve. Harvesting from mandibular ramus is more utilized than harvesting from symphisis since complications like significant change in the facial contours and post-operative sensory changes may occur in symphisis harvesting. Risk of neurovascular damage and difficult surgical access remain as disadvantages of harvesting from ramus, though [2, 41, 42].

3.1.2 Intraoral harvest from symphisis

Grafts harvested from mandibular symphisis is corticocancellous type. Due to anatomic limitations, blocks harvested from this site is shorter in length when compared to the blocks harvested from ramus. Maximal block dimensions are within the limits of mental foramina, apex of the anterior teeth and lower edge of the mandible. When harvesting from symphisis, osteotomies should be done 5 mm further from the apex of anterior teeth, mandibular lower edge and mental foramina. Easy surgical access and high amounts of osteoblasts make symphisis a preferable donor site. On the other hand, complications such as changes in the jaw contour, devitality of teeth and mental nerve damage may occur [34, 42].

3.2 Extraoral donor sites

Amount of bone volume harvested from intraoral donor sites is limited. Significantly greater graft volumes can be harvested from extraoral donor sites to reconstruct large size defects. Possible extraoral donor sites are calvaria, tibia, costae and iliac crest. Bone blocks obtained from extraoral donor sites tend to resorp faster than the blocks harvested intraorally. Therefore, greater volumes of bone should be harvested when reconstruction is planned with extraorally harvested bone blocks. Harvesting from extraoral donor sites have some major drawbacks such as increased morbidity at the donor site and requirement for patients to go under general anesthesia along with hospitalization afterwards [2, 5, 34].

Sbordone et al. evaluated resorption rates following iliac crest block bone grafting via CT images. In 6 years follow-up, %87 mean resorption rate is

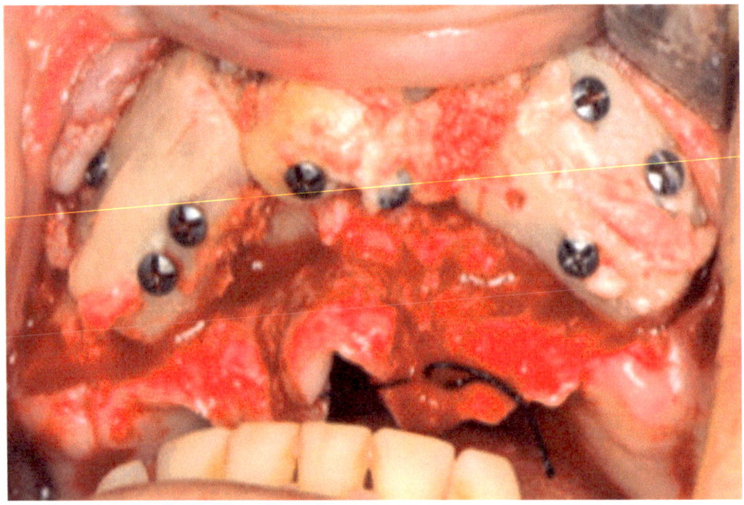

Figure 7.
Iliac block grafts fixated on the atrophic maxilla.

demonstrated at maxillary reconstruciton sites [43]. In a similar study conducted by Vermeeren et al., panoramic x-rays are evaluated for 5 years and resorption rates ranging between %44–50 are observed at sites grafted with block bones. Several studies report variety of resorption rates from %42 to %87 when autogenous block bone grafting is performed. Utilizing a collagen membrane along with autogenous block bone grafting is demonstrated to reduce resorption rates up to %25 (**Figure 7**) [44].

4. Alveolar ridge splitting

Alveolar ridge split is a common technique used in the presence of horizontally deficient alveolar ridges. Surgical procedure for this technique is initiated by one horizontal crestal osteotomy [45]. Piezosurgery, oscillating saws or diamond burs and chisels can be used for the initial osteotomy [2]. Different chisels of increasing width progressively create a gap between the buccal and palatinal/lingual plates afterwards. Interpositional grafting and/or immediate implant placement is oftenly applied to the created gap. This concept is based on the osseous plasticity of trabecular bone. Therefore, a 3- to 5 mm residual crest width is required for the procedure. Fractures may occur in ridges with lower width due to less presence of trabecular bone and less plasticity [46]. To gain greater amounts of new bone, vertical osteotomies may be added to the initial horizontal osteotomy. Another surgical concept of ridge splitting is the displacement of buccal plate by adding a second horizontal osteotomy apically to the initial horizontal osteotomy. In this concept, greenstick outfracture from the basal bone is created on purpose. If full-thickness flap is elevated, the plate should be fixed with screws to the palatinal/lingual plate. Partial-thickness flap is also preferred to keep periosteal vascularization when greenstick fracture is created [47, 48].

This procedure is indicated in cases presenting 3 to 5 mm bone width, with sufficient trabecular bone under the cortical layer. Two-stage ridge split is found to have high success rates up to %97 in terms of implant survival. Studies report 3 to 3.5 mm mean horizontal bone gain with this procedure [48]. Still, there are some drawbacks of this procedure: unpredictable results in severely atrophic crest where trabecular bone is not present, high risk of uncontrolled fractures when applied to narrow ridges (<3 mm), bone gain only in horizontal dimension [46].

5. Maxillary sinus augmentation

Maxillary sinus is one of the paranasal sinuses, located adjacent to posterior maxilla. It's an air-filled anatomical cavity, lined with a membrane called "Schneiderian Membrane". Bone resorption following tooth loss, in conjunction with maxillary sinus pneumatization, causes crestal atrophy in the maxillary posterior region. Maxillary sinus floor elevation provides enough bone height for implant placement in atrophic posterior maxilla. To elevate the Schneiderian Membrane, various techniques are developed. These techniques are classified in two main categories: lateral window approach and transalveolar approach.

5.1 Lateral window approach

This technique consists of preparing a window on buccal bone (also lateral wall of maxillary sinus) and elevating sinus membrane through the window. The superoinferior and anteroposterior borders of lateral window is determined depending on the location of maxillary sinus. Inferior border is usually 2 to 5 mm above the sinus floor to prevent any challenges during the infracturing. Once the lateral window is prepared and Schneiderian Membrane is elevated, various grafting materials can be added to the created space [49]. Barrier membranes are oftenly used to cover the bony window afterwards (**Figure 8**). Use of barrier membranes is reported to be more efficient than no membrane use in terms of implant survival rates [50]. In a clinical trial conducted by Garcia-Denche et al., no significant difference was found in lateral window approach with and without the use of membranes, though [51].

Lateral window approach is indicated when residual bone height is below 6 mm. Simultaneous implant placement may be applied when residual height is ≥4 mm. In cases presenting less than 4 mm of bone vertically, delayed implant placement is found to be safer [52]. Before proceeding to the surgery, a thorough medical examination is crucial to avoid possible complications. One of the most common complications in lateral window approach is bleeding during the flap elevation or preparation of lateral window. To avoid bleeding, inferior alveolar artery and posterior superior alveolar artery should be well examined, via radiographic images, in terms of location and possible anastomosis. Presence of septa should also be examined for a well-designed window preparation and for avoiding any membrane

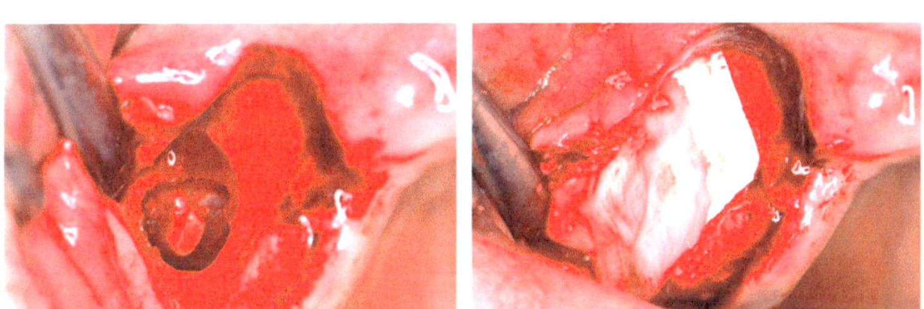

Figure 8.
Prepared lateral sinus access window (left) is closed by a resorbable barrier membrane (right) termed as the "open sinus lifting" or the "lateral window sinus lifting" technique.

perforations. Separate windows can be prepared, if necessary. Healthy Schneiderian Membrane is usually 1 mm thick. Thickness of the sinus membrane should be examined and pathological conditions must be treated before the surgery if present. In the presence of active sinus infection, neoplasmic lesions, uncontrolled diabetes, recurrent chronic sinusitis this technique is contraindicated [5, 49].

The augmented site is very well vascularized through surrounding sinus walls and Schneiderian Membrane, therefore it shows high success rates in terms of bone volume gain. Grafting is possible with various bone graft types. Graftless approach and grafting the site with highly degradable materials like collagen sponges or PRF is also possible but pneumatization of maxillary sinus and the required period for bone regeneration should be considered well enough before these approaches, since it's possible for membrane to collapse and decrease the bone gain [2, 49, 53].

5.2 Transalveolar approach

Comparing to lateral window approach, this technique is considered to be less invasive. It's indicated in cases with ≥6 mm residual bone height. In a retrospective clinical study by Rosen et al., implant survival rates were found to be higher where residual bone height is greater than 4 mm. This rate, which is 96% when the residual bone height is over 4 mm, decreases to 85.7% in the presence of bone height less than 4 mm [54]. In this approach, a pilot implant slot is created with a drill narrower than the final diameter of the implant. The pilot implant slot is prepared to a depth 1–2 mm from the sinus floor. Different osteotomes of increasing diameters and lengths are used to prepare the slot. It's recommended that the final osteotome has a diameter 0.5 mm less than the planned implant diameter. After the final osteotomy, dental implant is placed in the slot [49]. A group of researchers modified the technique by introducing bone grafts to osteotomy site before implant placement. This modification aims to increase bone amount between the implant and the sinus floor. However, Si et al. reported similar implant survival rates and no significant difference between grafted sites and nongrafted sites [55].

There are various modifications of membrane elevation in transalveolar approach: antral membrane baloon elevation, hydraulic sinus lift, hydrodynamic ultrasonic cavitation sinus lift, trephine core sinus lift and osseodensification.

Transalveolar approach is minimal invasive. Graft and membrane use is not compulsory with this technique and simultaneous implant placement is possible in eligible cases. On the contrary, full visualization of the surgical site is not possible

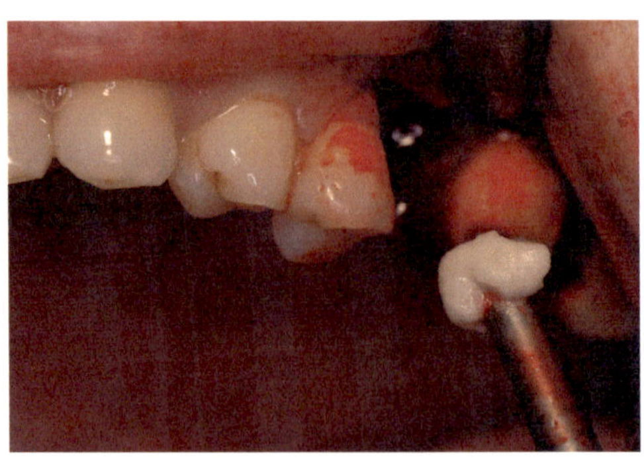

Figure 9.
Transcreastal osteotome technique used for the "closed sinus lifting" procedure. A bone graft was placed at the tip of the osteotome instrument for the prevention of the sinus membrane.

therefore possible complications, such as membrane perforations, may not be maintained well enough and intra-operatively (**Figure 9**), [46].

6. Distraction osteogenesis

Distraction osteogenesis is based on creating two bone segments by controlled osteotomies and gradually separating the segments to induce bone regeneration mechanism in between. In the surgical procedure, after full-thickness flap elevation and proper visualization of the site, fixation plates are temporarily adapted to the cortical bone. In this way, borders of osteotomy is determined. Following osteotomies, the distractor is fixed in the final position. Mobility of the transport segment is checked, then the device is put to initial passive position. Post-operative activation period is divided into three phases: latency, distraction, consolidation [2, 46, 56].

Latency: This protocol takes 5 to 7 days for a proper soft tissue healing. Distractor is not activated during this period to reduce the risk of wound dehiscence.

Distraction: Following latency, the distraction is activated by turning activation key at a rate of 0.5–1 mm per day. Transport segment is distracted from native bone vertically. Duration of distraction period depends on amount of bone needed.

Consolidation: Once the distraction is finalized, maturation of newly formed bone between the segments is expected for 8–12 weeks. Then the device is removed and implants are placed [2, 46].

Distraction osteogenesis can provide a bone gain of 5–15 mm vertically. Therefore it's safely indicated in vertical bone atrophies up to 15 mm [46]. In two clinical studies comparing autogenous bone block grafting and alveolar distraction osteogenesis (ADO), Bianchi et al. reported more bone gain in ADO group where Chiapasco et al. controversially reported no significant differences between the outcomes [56]. The procedure's contraindicated in cases presenting a thin knife-edge crest and insufficient bone amount to allow adequate anchorage. Patient co-operation during the distraction period is critical, treatment procedure should be thoroughly discussed with the patient before the initiation [46]. It is also a technique sensitive procedure, therefore it is recommended for experienced surgeons to practice [57].

There is no need for additional bone grafts and membranes with this technique. Gradual distraction helps soft tissue increase along with bone regeneration. There is minimal infection risk and resorption levels are low in the newly formed bone. In sites regenerated with distraction osteogenesis, implant survival rates are comparable with other techniques. Alveolar ridge is regenerated by it's own osteogenic and regenerative potential, therefore autogenous bone transplant is not needed in distraction osteogenesis. Functional and esthetic discomfort of distraction device in oral cavity remains as one of the disadvantages, though. A wide range of complications with a high incidence up to %76 is reported with distraction osteogenesis [2, 46, 58]. Chiapasco et al. stated 'change of distraction vector' as the most frequent complication. Premature consolidation, insufficient distraction, resorption of transport segment and fractures of native bone, the transport segment or the device is among the possible complications [59].

7. Conclusions

This chapter reviewed various alveolar ridge augmentation techniques in implant dentistry in general aspect. Alveolar ridge augmentation procedures are advanced surgical interventions. Success of these interventions depend on many factors such as the surgeon's experience, preferred technique, materials in use, patient's medical condition, defect topography and patient co-operation. With variety of factors affecting the outcome, it's hard to choose one technique over other. Guided bone regeneration and autogenous block bone grafting are two of the well-documented and safely applicable augmentation techniques. Both these techniques have challenging learning curves and require advanced skills in practice therefore following the evidence-based principles is critical for achieving successful outcomes.

Conflict of interest

The author declares no conflict of interest.

Thanks

Yeşim Aytekin Yaşar, the beloved sister of Melike Aytekin, is acknowledged for her support and encourage to her sister in the preparation of this chapter.

Author details

Melike Aytekin* and Volkan Arisan
Department of Oral Implantology, Faculty of Dentistry, Istanbul University, Istanbul, Turkey

*Address all correspondence to: aytekin.melike@gmail.com

References

[1] Liu J, Kerns DG. Mechanisms of guided bone regeneration: a review. The Open Dentistry Journal. 2014;**16**:56-65. DOI: 10.2174/1874210601408010056

[2] Tolstunov L, Hamrick JFE, Broumand V, Shilo D, Rachmiel A. Bone augmentation techniques for horizontal and vertical alveolar ridge deficiency in oral implantology. Oral and Maxillofacial Surgery Clinics. 2019;*31*(2):163-191. DOI: 10.1016/j.coms.2019.01.005

[3] Pikos, Michael A., Miron, Richard J. Bone Augmentation in Implant Dentistry: A Step-by-Step Guide to Predictable Alveolar Ridge and Sinus Grafting. Quintessence; 2019. 272 p. ISBN: 978-0867158250

[4] Aghaloo TL, Moy PK. Which hard tissue augmentation techniques are the most successful in furnishing bony support for implant placement? The International Journal of Oral & Maxillofacial Implants. 2007;**22** (Suppl):49-70

[5] Misch CE. Contemporary Implant Dentistry. St. Louis: Mosby-Year Book, Inc; 1993

[6] Probst A, Spiegel HU. Cellular mechanisms of bone repair. Journal of Investigative Surgery. 1997;**10**:77-86

[7] Gultekin BA, Cansız E, Yalçın S. Ridge Augmentation Techniques in Preprosthetic Implant. Surgery. 2016

[8] Urban IA, Monje A. Guided Bone Regeneration in Alveolar Bone Reconstruction. Oral and Maxillofacial Surgery Clinics. 2019;*31*(2):331-338

[9] Schenk RK, Buser D, Hardwick WR, et al. Healing pattern of bone regeneration in membrane-protected defects: a histologic study in the canine mandible. The International Journal of Oral & Maxillofacial Implants. 1994;**9**:13-29

[10] Urban IA, Jovanovic SA, Lozada JL. Vertical ridge augmentation using guided bone regeneration (GBR) in three clinical scenarios prior to implant placement: a retrospective study of 35 patients 12 to 72 months after loading. The International Journal of Oral & Maxillofacial Implants. 2009;**24**:502-510

[11] Liu J, Kerns DG. Mechanisms of guided bone regeneration: a review. The Open Dentistry Journal. 2014;**16**:56-65. DOI: 10.2174/1874210601408010056

[12] Benic GI, Hämmerle CH. Horizontal bone augmentation by means of guided bone regeneration. Periodontol 2000. 2014;66:13-40. doi: 10.1111/prd.12039.

[13] Gultekin BA, Siyli GZA. Hard Tissue Regeneration Treatment Protocols in Contemporary Oral Surgery. Tissue Regeneration. 2018;**141**

[14] Owens KW, Yukna RA. Collagen membrane resorption in dogs: a comparative study. Implant Dentistry. 2001;**10**:49-58

[15] Miller N, Penaud J, Foliguet B, Membre H, Ambrosini P, Plombas M. Resorption rates of 2 commercially available bioresorbable membranes. A histomorphometric study in a rabbit model. Journal of Clinical Periodontology. 1996;**23**:1051-1059

[16] Rothamel D, Schwarz F, Fienitz T, Smeets R, Dreiseidler T, Ritter L, et al. Biocompatibility and biodegradation of a native porcine pericardium membrane: results of in vitro and in vivo examinations. The International Journal of Oral & Maxillofacial Implants. 2012; **27**:146

[17] Ausenda F, Rasperini G, Acunzo R, Gorbunkova A, Pagni G. New

Perspectives in the Use of Biomaterials for Periodontal Regeneration. Materials (Basel). 2019;12(13):2197. Published 2019 Jul 8. doi:10.3390/ma12132197

[18] Ronda M, Rebaudi A, Torelli L, Stacchi C. Expanded vs. dense polytetrafluoroethylene membranes in vertical ridge augmentation around dental implants: a prospective randomized controlled clinical trial. Clinical Oral Implants Research. 2014;**25**(7):859-866

[19] Jensen SS, Terheyden H. Bone augmentation proced in localized defects in the alveolar ridge : Clinical results with different bone grafts and bone- substitute materials. International Journal of Oral & Maxillofacial Implants. 2009;**24**:218-236

[20] Jovanovic SA, Nevins M. Bone formation utilizing titanium- reinforced barrier mem- branes. The International Journal of Periodontics & Restorative Dentistry. 1995;**15**:56-69

[21] Urist MR. Bone morphogenetic protein: the molecularization of skeletal system development. Journal of Bone and Mineral Research. 1997;*12*(3):343-346

[22] Zakhary IE, El-Mekkawi HA, Elsalanty ME. Alveolar ridge augmentation for implant fixation: status review. Oral surgery, oral medicine, oral pathology and oral radiology. 2012;*114*(5):S179-S189

[23] Tolstunov L. Horizontal Alveolar Ridge Augmentation in Implant Dentistry: A Surgical Manual. John Wiley & Sons; 2015

[24] Listgarten GS. Periodontics. Sixth ed. ;**1998**:860-879

[25] Wessing B, Lettner S, Zechner W. Guided Bone Regeneration with Collagen Membranes and Particulate Graft Materials: A Systematic Review and Meta-Analysis. The International Journal of Oral & Maxillofacial Implants. 2018;**33**(1):87-100. DOI: 10.11607/jomi.5461

[26] Mendoza-Azpur G, de la Fuente A, Chavez E, Valdivia E, Khouly I. Horizontal ridge augmentation with guided bone regeneration using particulate xenogenic bone substitutes with or without autogenous block grafts: A randomized controlled trial. Clinical Implant Dentistry and Related Research. 2019;**21**(4):521-530

[27] Bouler JM, Pilet P, Gauthier O, Verron E. Biphasic calcium phosphate ceramics for bone reconstruction: A review of biological response. Acta Biomaterialia. 2017;**53**:1-12. DOI: 10.1016/j.actbio.2017.01.076

[28] Choi BH, Zhu SJ, Kim BY, Huh JY, Lee SH, Jung JH. Effect of platelet rich plasma con- centration on the viability and proliferation of alveolar bone cells: An in vitro study. International Journal of Oral and Maxillofacial Surgery. 2005;S:420-424

[29] Raja SV, Naidue ME. Platelet rich fibrin: Evolution of a scond geneation platelet concen- trate. Indian Journal of Dental Research. 2007;S:42-46

[30] Paulla N, Wolter T, Morcowicz M. Platelet rich plasma in burns. Burns. 2009;S:4-8

[31] Kathleen ML, Dardık A. Platelet rich plasma: Support for its use in wound healing. Yale Journal of Biology and Medicine. 2010:1-9

[32] Dohan DM, Choukroun J, Diss A, Dohan SL, Dohan AJ, Mouhyi J, et al. Platelet rich fibrin (PRF): A second generation platelet concentrate. Part II: Leucocyte activation : A new feature for platelet concentrates? Oral Surgery, Oral Medicine, Oral Pathology, Oral Radiology, and Endodontics. 2006;**1011**:51-55

[33] Nakashima M, Reddi AH. The application of bone morphogenetic proteins to dental tissue engineering. Nature Biotechnology. 2003;**21**:1025-1032

[34] Idrontino, G., & Valente, N. A. (2016). Intraoral and extraoral autologous bone block graft techniques: A review of the recent literature. International Journal of Contemporary Dental & Medical Reviews, 2016.

[35] Aloy-Prósper A, Peñarrocha-Oltra D, Peñarrocha-Diago MA, Peñarrocha-Diago M. The outcome of intraoral onlay block bone grafts on alveolar ridge augmentations: a systematic review. Medicina oral, patologia oral y cirugia bucal. 2015;**20**(2):e251

[36] Jensen AT, Jensen SS, Worsaae N. Complications related to bone augmentation procedures of localized defects in the alveolar ridge. A retrospective clinical study. *Oral and maxillofacial surgery*. 2016;*20*(2):115-122

[37] Chappuis V, Cavusoglu Y, Buser D, von Arx T. Lateral ridge augmentation using autogenous block grafts and guided bone regeneration: A 10-year prospective case series study. Clinical Implant Dentistry and Related Research. 2017;**19**(1):85-96

[38] McAllister BS, Haghighat K. Bone augmentation techniques. Journal of Periodontology. 2007;*78*(3):377-396

[39] Gultekin BA, Cansiz E, Borahan MO. Clinical and 3-dimensional radiographic evaluation of autogenous iliac block bone grafting and guided bone regeneration in patients with atrophic maxilla. Journal of Oral and Maxillofacial Surgery. 2017;**75**(4):709-722

[40] Nkenke E, Neukam FW. Autogenous bone harvesting and grafting in advanced jaw resorption: morbidity, resorption and implant survival. Eur J Oral Implantol. 2014;**7**(Suppl 2):S203-S217

[41] Cunha G, Rocha AFL, Pereira Filho VA, Gabrielli MFR, Gabrielli MAC. Atrophic maxilla reconstruction with autogenous iliac graft and guided dental implants. Journal of Craniofacial Surgery. 2018;**29**(8):2218-2219

[42] Sethi A, Kaus T, Cawood JI, Plaha H, Boscoe M, Sochor P. Onlay bone grafts from iliac crest: a retrospective analysis. International Journal of Oral and Maxillofacial Surgery. 2020;**49**(2): 264-271

[43] Sbordone C, Toti P, Guidetti F, Califano L, Santoro A, Sbordone L. Volume changes of iliac crest autogenous bone grafts after vertical and horizontal alveolar ridge augmen- tation of atrophic maxillas and mandibles: a 6-year computerized tomographic follow- up. Journal of Oral and Maxillofacial Surgery. 2012;**70**:2559-2565. DOI: 10.1016/j.joms.2012.07.040.

[44] Vermeeren JI, Wismeijer D, van Waas MA. One-step reconstruction of the severely resorbed mandible with onlay bone grafts and endosteal implants. A 5-year follow-up. International Journal of Oral and Maxillofacial Surgery. 1996;**25**:112-115

[45] Elnayef B, Monje A, Lin G, Gargallo-Albiol J, Chan HL, Wang HL, et al. Alveolar Ridge Split on Horizontal Bone Augmentation: A Systematic Review. The International Journal of Oral & Maxillofacial Implants. 2015;**30**:596-606. DOI: 10.11607/jomi.4051.

[46] Malet J, Mora F, Bouchard P. Implant Dentistry at a Glance. Wiley-Blackwell; 2012. 144 p. ISBN: 978-1-4443-3744-0.

[47] Starch-Jensen T, Becktor JP. Maxillary Alveolar Ridge Expansion with Split-Crest Technique Compared with Lateral Ridge Augmentation with Autogenous Bone Block Graft: a

Systematic Review. J Oral Maxillofac Res. 2019;10(4):e2. Published 2019 Dec 30. doi:10.5037/jomr.2019.10402

[48] Agabiti I, Botticelli D. Two-Stage Ridge Split at Narrow Alveolar Mandibular Bone Ridges. J Oral Maxillofac Surg. 2017;75(10):2115.e1-2115.e12. doi:10.1016/j.joms.2017.05.015

[49] Mohan N, Wolf J, Dym H. Maxillary sinus augmentation. Dental Clinics of North America. 2015;**59**(2):375-388. DOI: 10.1016/j.cden.2014.10.001

[50] Tonetti MS, Hämmerle CH; European Workshop on Periodontology Group C. Advances in bone augmentation to enable dental implant placement: Consensus Report of the Sixth European Workshop on Periodontology. Journal of Clinical Periodontology 2008;35(8 Suppl):168-172. doi:10.1111/j.1600-051X.2008.01268.x

[51] García-Denche JT, Wu X, Martinez PP, et al. Membranes over the lateral window in sinus augmentation procedures: a two-arm and split-mouth randomized clinical trials. Journal of Clinical Periodontology. 2013;**40**(11):1043-1051. DOI: 10.1111/jcpe.12153

[52] Zitzmann NU, Schärer P. Sinus elevation procedures in the resorbed posterior maxilla. Comparison of the crestal and lateral approaches. Oral Surgery, Oral Medicine, Oral Pathology, Oral Radiology, and Endodontics. 1998;**85**(1):8-17. DOI: 10.1016/s1079-2104(98)90391-2

[53] Ting M, Rice JG, Braid SM, Lee CYS, Suzuki JB. Maxillary Sinus Augmentation for Dental Implant Rehabilitation of the Edentulous Ridge: A Comprehensive Overview of Systematic Reviews. Implant Dentistry. 2017;**26**(3):438-464. DOI: 10.1097/ID.0000000000000606

[54] Rosen PS, Summers R, Mellado JR, et al. The bone-added osteotome sinus floor elevation technique: multicenter retrospective report of consecutively treated patients. The International Journal of Oral & Maxillofacial Implants. 1999;**14**(6):853-858

[55] Si MS, Zhuang LF, Gu YX, Mo JJ, Qiao SC, Lai HC. Osteotome sinus floor elevation with or without grafting: a 3-year randomized controlled clinical trial. Journal of Clinical Periodontology. 2013;**40**(4):396-403. DOI: 10.1111/jcpe.12066

[56] Toledano-Serrabona J, Sánchez-Garcés MÁ, Sánchez-Torres A, Gay-Escoda C. Alveolar distraction osteogenesis for dental implant treatments of the vertical bone atrophy: A systematic review. Med Oral Patol Oral Cir Bucal. 2019;24(1):e70-e75. Published 2019 Jan 1. doi:10.4317/medoral.22750

[57] Liou JW, Chen KT. Intraoral Distraction of Segmental Osteotomies and Miniscrews in Management of Alveolar Cleft. Seminars in Orthodontics. 2009;**15**:257-267

[58] Sahoo NK, Issar Y, Thakral A. Mandibular Distraction Osteogenesis. The Journal of Craniofacial Surgery. 2019;**30**(8):e743-e746. DOI: 10.1097/SCS.0000000000005753

[59] Chiapasco M, Consolo U, Bianchi A, Ronchi P. Alveolar distraction osteogenesis for the correction of vertically deficient edentulous ridges: a multicenter prospective study on humans. The International Journal of Oral & Maxillofacial Implants. 2004;**19**(3):399-407

Chapter 9

A Review of Maxillofacial Rehabilitation Using Osseointegrated Implants in Oncological Patients: Buttress Implant Concept

Leandro Díez-Suárez, Vicente González-Cardín, Antonio Gómez-Pedraza and Martín Granados-García

Abstract

Cancer leaves important consequences in the shape, function and esthetics of the patient, especially when it is cancer of the oral cavity or upper aero-digestive tract. Although reconstruction with local and microvascular flaps is sometimes a viable option, maxillofacial rehabilitation with osseointegrated implants is a well-reported treatment alternative with a high success rate. The main advantages in this modality of rehabilitation are the decrease in biological and economic costs, simplifying the management of these defects by reducing surgical intervention, hospitalization time, postoperative morbidity and treatment time. There are several classification systems; however, there is no classification system that has accurately described the maxillofacial defect under a surgical, prosthetic and reconstructive approach with osseointegrated implants. The purpose of this study is to guide professionals in decision-making for maxillofacial rehabilitation using osseointegrated implants located in the anatomical buttresses of the maxillofacial region.

Keywords: dental implants, anatomical buttress, maxillectomy defects, maxillofacial rehabilitation, prosthodontic reconstruction

1. Introduction

In 2018, The Global Cancer Statistics reported just over 18 million new cases worldwide. Lip and oral cavity cancer is ranked 18th with 354,864 new cases (2.0%) and 177,384 deaths (1.9%). However, if we analyze the main cancers that affect the upper digestive tract (salivary glands, hypopharynx, oropharynx, nasopharynx, larynx, lip, and oral cavity), we obtain approximately 887,659 new cases (4.9%) of cancers that could leave important sequelae in the maxillofacial region [1].

Maxillectomy is defined as the partial or total surgical removal of the maxilla and was designed as a surgical treatment for tumors that affect the middle third of the face. During oncological ablative surgery complex maxillofacial defects result that involve the loss of anatomical structures such as dental elements, facial cavities, sense organs, bone tissue and facial soft tissue. Although reconstruction with local and microvascular flaps is sometimes a viable alternative, maxillofacial rehabilitation with osseointegrated implants has been a well-reported treatment with a high success rate [2].

Various techniques and anatomical locations have been described in the facial region for the placement of osseointegrated implants and its reason is based on the bone buttress where a skeletal anchorage is possible to support the functional load of the implants. In general, maxillofacial rehabilitation with osseointegrated implants uses anchors in the zygomatic, pterygoid, nasomaxillary and alveolar zones [3–5].

2. Buttress implant concept and classification

Based on the anatomical zones of the bony buttresses of the facial middle third, we designed a classification system that allows determining the therapeutic options where the placement and functional loading of osseointegrated implants is feasible: zone I or alveolar, zone II or nasomaxillary, zone III or zygomatic, zone IV or pterygoid (**Figure 1**).

2.1 Zone I/maxillary alveolar buttress

2.1.1 Tilted and axially positioned implants

The use of endosseous osseointegrated implants was introduced to North America in 1982. At that conference, Branemark presented the data from 15 years of work, which was highly evidence-based with long-term clinical follow-up findings setting the guidelines for contemporary implantology [6].

Currently implantology has improved considerably; dental implants have incorporated advances in their anatomy, surface and types of connections, achieving a higher success rate and predictable results [7, 8].

Implants angled between 30 and 45° were described as an alternative surgical technique in order to avoid nearby anatomical structures or to achieve an adjacent bone position. Thus, we avoid advanced bone regeneration procedures and minimize the cantilever of prosthetic rehabilitation [9].

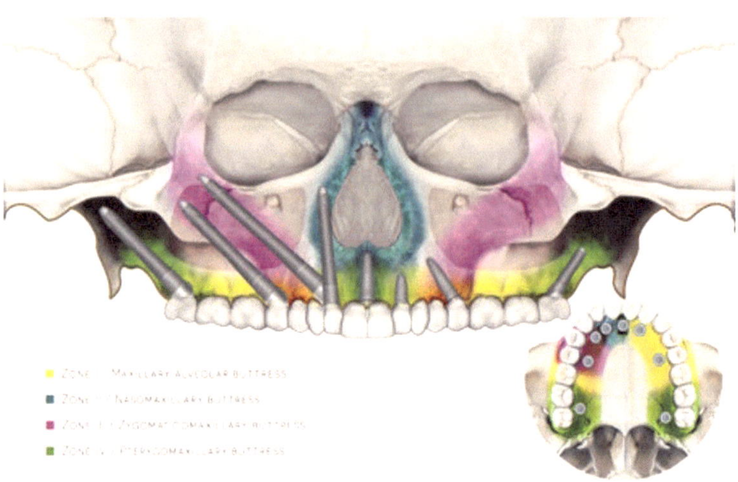

Figure 1.
Anatomical zones of the bony buttresses of the facial middle third and placement of osseointegrated implants with their positions in the prosthetic arch.

2.1.2 Nasopalatine implants

In 1994 Scher. describes the use of the nasopalatine canal as a receptor site for a dental implant, since then controlled studies have been carried out that confirm its viability for the functional load of osseointegrated implants [10].

Peñarrocha et al. treated 13 patients with 78 osseointegrated implants in the rehabilitation of the atrophic maxilla. Of 78 implants, 13 were implanted in the nasopalatine canal, 6 patients had reversible sensory alteration, and 2 implants failed in healthy patients, yielding a success rate of 84.6% [11].

Occasionally, when performing a partial maxillectomy, bone is available throughout the Maxillary alveolar buttress. In these cases, it is possible to use conventional dental implants anchored even in contralateral anatomical structures.

2.2 Zone II/nasomaxillary buttress

2.2.1 Nasomaxillary implants

Although the term "Nasomaxillary implant" has not been defined in the Glossary of Oral and Maxillofacial Implants (GOMI) [12]. We define it as "Implant placement through the alveolar process and into the nasomaxillary buttress".

The nasomaxillary buttress has been well described in facial trauma as it is a key anatomic zone in the reconstruction of fractures of the middle third. This area offers a cortical bone suitable for the anchorage and functional load of osseointegrated implants. However, there are few implant-oriented anatomical studies and some are anthropometric studies [13–16].

Some authors have described the placement of posterior tilted implants between 30 and 45° that reach an apical anchorage in the nasomaxillary buttress [9, 17, 18]. However, this type of implant is not frankly a nasomaxillary implant because they are retained from an apical portion and are not strictly into the buttress as in the case of a long implant with an axial orientation.

Nasomaxillary implants can be used as an anchorage point in a location anterior to the prosthetic arch. With this, we achieve anterior stability and the reduction of work forces in posterior implants.

2.3 Zone III/zygomaticomaxillary buttress

2.3.1 Zygomatic implants

In 1998 Dr. P. I Branemark described zygomatic implants as a bone anchorage alternative with a design between 30 and 52.5 mm long that are inserted into the body of the malar bone [19]. Since then, Branemark and other authors have described various surgical techniques and approaches for zygomatic implant placement that could be used to rehabilitate atrophic jaws or in patients with partial or total maxillectomy [20–22].

Scott et al. rehabilitated 28 patients after undergoing rhinectomy for malignant pathological processes, a total of 56 zygomatic implants were used as retainers of maxillofacial prostheses, 1 failed after radiotherapy having a success rate of 98% in 15 years [4].

In general, most authors agree that zygomatic implants are more than 95% successful [23] and in radiated patients the success rate of implants is highly variable with a range between 72 and 98% [2].

Zygomatic implants offer adequate bone quality and quantity. Sometimes when the maxillectomy is extensive, it compromises the malar bone. Performing regenerative procedures with autografts or xenografts are a viable option to improve site conditions.

2.4 Zone IV/pterygomaxillary buttress

2.4.1 Pterygomaxillary implants

Tulasne and Tessier in 1989 were the first to describe the technique for the placement of pterygoid implants [24]. This technique wanted to resolve the difficulties caused by the presence of the maxillary sinus and the poor characteristics of the bone in the maxillary tuberosity.

Pterygoid implants are implants between 15 and 20 mm long that allow a bone anchorage of up to 9 mm in the pterygoid process [25]. However, in the maxilectomized patient this length may vary because the posterior segment of the maxilla is not found.

Araujo et al. in 2019 performed a systematic review from January 1995 to January 2018. A total of 634 patients received 1893 pterygoid implants, with a 10-year survival rate of 94.85%.

Pterygoid implants are a viable option and if their main advantage is to decrease the prosthetic distal cantilever [26].

3. Buttress implant concept: advantages and disadvantages

Maxillofacial reconstruction with osseointegrated implants placed in bony buttresses is indicated in patients who have suffered loss of mid-facial anatomical structures due to benign and malignant pathological processes, trauma, and severe maxillary atrophy.

There are few contraindications to the use of osseointegrated implants and they are mostly relative. Their reason is that they decrease the success rate compared to implantation in healthy patients. The most important contraindications suggest bone healing disorders such as bisphosphonate treatment, radiotherapy, chemotherapy and active infection. However, for each situation there are protocols that help maintain a high success rate and some of them are discussed in this chapter [20, 23, 27].

The main advantages in this type of rehabilitation are the decrease in the number of reconstructive surgeries, avoiding the use of donor sites and a shorter hospital stay. By performing a single-phase reconstruction, the patient recovers the phonation, swallowing and chewing lost due to the oncological defect. in addition, the patients present a timely and less morbid treatment compared to local and microvascular grafts. To achieve these results, prosthetically guided reconstruction is key [28].

4. Virtual prosthetic and surgical planning

Three-dimensional (3D) planning in oral and maxillofacial surgery has become a standard in the treatment of multiple conditions of the facial region. Multiple Programs have been designed to perform 3D virtual planning and surgery in the reconstruction with osseointegrated implants (DTX Studio Implant®, SIMPLANT®, DDS-pro®, 3Shape Dental System®). Most of them are equipped with numerous software complements that allow the preparation of surgical guides and prosthetic reconstructions with different attachments through CAD/CAM [29].

Some of the multiple advantages offered by 3D virtual surgery are: simulating different approaches and types of procedures, avoiding damage to neurovascular and anatomical structures, reducing operating time and improving postoperative recovery, reducing complications and obtaining more predictable results.

For preoperative evaluation and planning, a CT scan of the head and neck is the Gold standard [3, 23]. The planning of the placement of osseointegrated implants must be prosthetically guided. This means that planning must precede the surgical act of implant placement and these must be located where it best suits prosthetic rehabilitation and biomechanical demands. The objective should be a surgical and prosthetic planning with at least four osseointegrated implants with their distributed emergencies in a polygonal manner over the prosthetic arch. In this way, we were able to tripodize and stabilize the prosthetic reconstruction in the face of the functional demands of chewing (**Figure 2**) [28, 30].

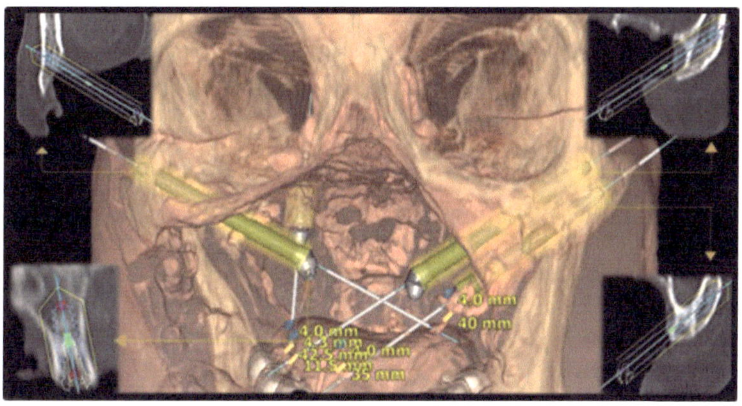

Figure 2.
3-dimensional computed prosthetic and surgical planning and bone availability in the peri-implant anatomical zone.

5. Simulated surgery in stereolithographic biomodels

Stereolithography is a solid three-dimensional prototype obtained through the processing of data obtained from computed tomography or magnetic resonance imaging. In recent years, stereolithographic manufacturing has made great strides in the quality, resolution, and precision of manufactured parts and is becoming increasingly important in medicine and surgery [31].

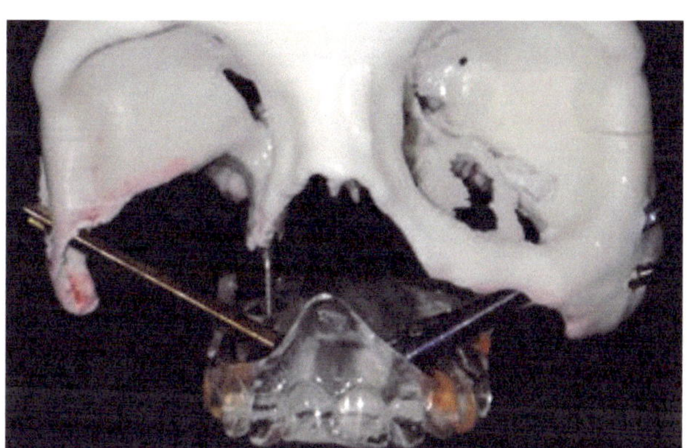

Figure 3.
Simulated surgery in stereolithographic biomodel. Zygomatic and Pterygomaxillary implants placed in the planned positions.

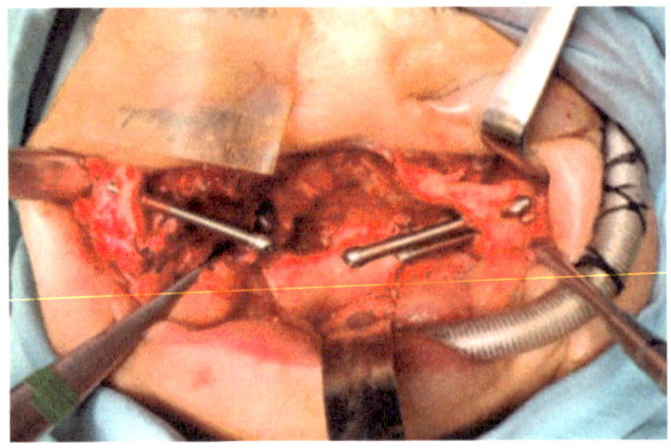

Figure 4.
Photograph of surgical field after placement of zygomatic and Pterygomaxillary implants.

Three-dimensional printing has been used to produce anatomical models, surgical guides and templates, implants, and molds. The main advantages include: the possibility of preoperative planning, the precision of the process used and the time saved in the operating room. However, other studies report inconsistency in precision and additional costs in treatment [32].

The maxillofacial reconstruction with osseointegrated implants simulated in a biomodel, allows to determine the lengths and final positions of the implants, prepare the surgeon for the surgical procedure and minimize the possibilities of errors favoring the results of the treatment (**Figures 3** and **4**).

6. Prosthetic and facial reconstruction

Oral and facial deformity can cause functional and psychological deterioration in oncological patients. The aims of prosthodontic reconstruction are the rehabilitation of the shape, function and esthetics of the lost anatomical structures by means of artificial substitutes. The main facial subunits that require reconstruction due to malignant pathological processes involve the ear, forehead, eyes and brow, nose, check, lips and chin [33].

Currently, there are multiple workflows where they combine conventional prosthetic preparation with the use of facial scanners and custom 3D impressions

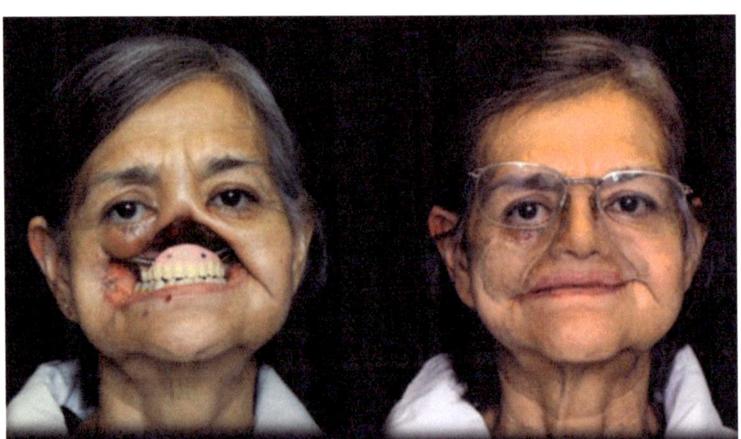

Figure 5.
Photograph showing implant-supported obturator placed and final photograph.

that allow the direct or indirect manufacture of definitive maxillofacial prostheses from conventional silicone [34, 35].

The main advantage with dental prosthodontic reconstruction is the adaptation of a retained implant obturator that allows a posterior palatal seal. With this, most patients successfully recover phonation, swallowing, and chewing function. Artificial facial prostheses allow us to better characterize the demanding anatomy of the face. In most cases, the retention of facial prostheses occurs when copying the anatomical defect, on other occasions magnetized attachments can be used in prosthetic reconstruction or protective glasses that also improve the characterization of the face (**Figure 5**).

7. Radiotherapy treatment and implants

In early clinical stages, surgery is the first decision. However, adjuvant radiotherapy is sometimes indicated in cases of close excision margins (<5 mm), involved (<1 mm), and in suspicion or confirmation of lymph node metastasis with or without extracapsular extension [36]. In general, radiation therapy includes conventional radiation therapy or intensity modulated radiation therapy (IMRT). The latter is more convenient by precisely targeting radiation to a specific area and reducing the dose to nearby anatomical structures such as malar bone, grafts, implants, salivary glands, eyes, and spinal cord [37].

Schiegnitz's study suggests that radiation negatively affects implant survival, but there is no statistically significant difference in survival when implants are inserted 12 months before or after radiation therapy [38]. Other authors have shown favorable results. With implantation at least 6 weeks before radiotherapy since there is a surgical area with less hypoxia, hypovascularity and hypocellularity [27, 39] (**Figure 6**).

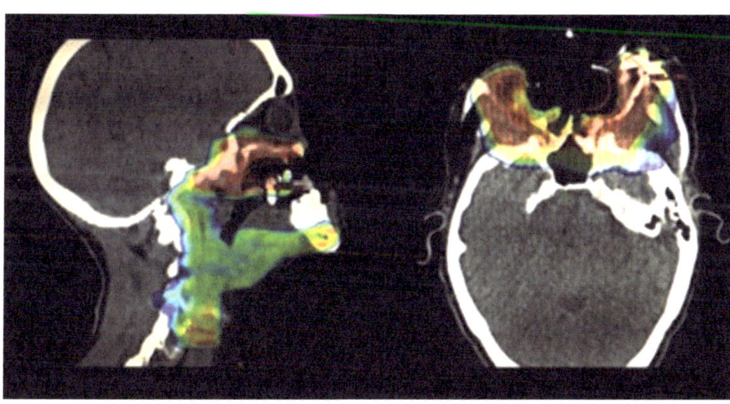

Figure 6.
Histogram showing trajectories, dose and volume used for adjuvant radiotherapy.

8. Chemotherapy treatment and implants

Systemic antineoplastic therapy includes induction, neoadjuvant, adjuvant, and palliative therapy [40]. The survival rate of osseointegrated implants in the patient with antineoplastic and antiangiogenic therapy has not yet been elucidated. Controlled animal studies have shown negative effects on the osseointegration process with chemotherapeutic regimens with cisplatin, bevacizumab and sunitinib [41–43]. However, retrospective studies in humans have reported that chemotherapy has no detrimental effects on the osseointegration and functional stability of dental implants. The success rates reported by these studies were 97.6 and 99.1% [44–46].

9. Conclusion

The placement of osseointegrated implants in anatomical buttresses of the upper jaw is a predictable treatment with a high success rate. By reconstructing the lost anatomical structures with artificial substitutes, a better characterization of the face is achieved and an important esthetic defect is covered with acceptable results.

The main advantages in this modality of reconstruction include the decrease in surgical times, hospital stay and postoperative morbidity. By rehabilitating phonation, swallowing and masticatory function, we improve the quality of life and social reintegration of the oncological patient.

Currently, technological advances point to the development in the design of customized implants; however, controlled studies are required to evaluate the use and behavior of these implants in the different scenarios presented by the oncological patient.

Acknowledgements

To the National Cancer Institute - Mexico City and the head and neck medical department for the comprehensive treatment of oncological patients. To Dr. Víctor Felipe Orduña López for the joint treatment.

Conflict of interest

There are no conflicts of interest to declare.

Ethical approval

Institutional approval was not required.

Author details

Leandro Díez-Suárez[1,3]*, Vicente González-Cardín[2], Antonio Gómez-Pedraza[3] and Martín Granados-García[3]

1 Oral and Maxillofacial Surgeon Department, National Autonomous University of Mexico UNAM, Mexico City, Mexico

2 Head and Neck Prosthodontist Department, National Cancer Institute, Mexico City, Mexico

3 Head and Neck Surgery Department, National Cancer Institute, Mexico City, Mexico

*Address all correspondence to: ledisuar@gmail.com

References

[1] Bray F, Ferlay J, Soerjomataram I, Siegel RL, Torre LA, Jemal A. Global cancer statistics 2018: GLOBOCAN estimates of incidence and mortality worldwide for 36 cancers in 185 countries. CA: A Cancer Journal for Clinicians. 2018;**68**(6):394-424

[2] Gómez-Pedraza A, González-Cardín V, Díez-Suárez L, Herrera-Villalva M. Maxillofacial rehabilitation with zygomatic implants in an oncologic patient: A case report. Journal of Oral and Maxillofacial Surgery. 2020;**78**(4): 547-556. DOI: 10.1016/j.joms.2019.10.006

[3] Pellegrino G, Tarsitano A, Basile F, Pizzigallo A, Marchetti C. Computer-aided rehabilitation of maxillary oncological defects using zygomatic implants: A defect-based classification. Journal of Oral and Maxillofacial Surgery. 2015;**73**(12):2446.e1-2446.e11. DOI: 10.1016/j.joms.2015.08.020

[4] Scott N, Kittur MA, Evans PL, Dovgalski L, Hodder SC. The use of zygomatic implants for the retention of nasal prosthesis following rhinectomy: The Morriston experience. International Journal of Oral & Maxillofacial Surgery. 2016;**45**(8):1044-1048. DOI: 10.1016/j.ijom.2016.01.020

[5] Vrielinck L, Politis C, Schepers S, Pauwels M, Naert I. Image-based planning and clinical validation of zygoma and pterygoid implant placement in patients with severe bone atrophy using customized drill guides. Preliminary results from a prospective clinical follow-up study. International Journal of Oral and Maxillofacial Surgery. 2003;**32**(1):7-14

[6] Block MS. Dental implants: The last 100 years. Journal of Oral and Maxillofacial Surgery. 2018;**76**(1):11-26

[7] Ogle OE. Implant surface material, design, and osseointegration. Dental Clinics of North America. 2015;**59**(2):505-520. DOI: 10.1016/j.cden.2014.12.003

[8] Smeets R, Stadlinger B, Schwarz F, Beck-Broichsitter B, Jung O, Precht C, et al. Impact of dental implant surface modifications on osseointegration. BioMed Research International. 2016;**2016**:6285620. DOI: 10.1155/2016/6285620

[9] Soto-Peñaloza D, Zaragozí-Alonso R, Peñarrocha-Diago M, Peñarrocha-Diago M. The all-on-four treatment concept: Systematic review. Journal of Clinical and Experimental Dentistry. 2017;**9**(3):e474–e488

[10] Scher E. Use of the incisive canal as a recipient site for root form implants: Preliminary clinical reports. Implant Dentistry. 1994;**3**:38-41

[11] Peñarrocha D, Candel E, Guirado JL, Canullo LPM. Implants placed in the nasopalatine canal to rehabilitate severely atrophic maxillae: A retrospective study with long follow-up. The Journal of Oral Implantology. 2014;**40**(6):699-706

[12] Laney W. Oral and endorsing organizations. The International Journal of Oral & Maxillofacial Implants. 2017;**32**:Gi-G200

[13] McCollum MA. Nasomaxillary remodeling and facial form in robust australopithecus: A reassessment. Journal of Human Evolution. 2008;**54**(1):2-14

[14] Hwang TS, Song J, Yoon H, Cho BP, Kang HS. Morphometry of the nasal bones and piriform apertures in Koreans. Annals of Anatomy. 2005;**187**(4):411-414

[15] Adnot J, Desbarats C, Joly LM, Trost O. Nasomaxillary fracture:

Retrospective review of 11 consecutive patients and literature review. Journal of Stomatology, Oral and Maxillofacial Surgery. 2019;**120**(6):534-539. DOI: 10.1016/j.jormas.2019.03.003

[16] Hsiao S, Cheng J, Tseng Y. ScienceDirect nasomaxillary and mandibular bone growth in primary school girls aged 7 to 12 years. The Internet Journal of Dental Science. 2020;**xxxx**:3-8. DOI: 10.1016/j.jds.2020.03.010

[17] Jensen OT. Dental extraction, immediate placement of dental implants, and immediate function. Oral and Maxillofacial Surgery Clinics of North America. 2015;**27**(2):273-282. DOI: 10.1016/j.coms.2015.01.008

[18] Jensen OT, Adams MW, Butura C, Galindo DF. Maxillary V-4: Four implant treatment for maxillary atrophy with dental implants fixed apically at the vomer-nasal crest, lateral pyriform rim, and zygoma for immediate function. Report on 44 patients followed from 1 to 3 years. Journal of Prosthetic Dentistry. 2015;**114, 6**:810-817. DOI: 10.1016/j.prosdent.2014.11.018

[19] Branemark P. Surgery Fixture Installation: Zygomaticus Fixture Clinical Procedures. 1st ed. Gotemburgo, Suecia: Nobel Bio- care, AB; 1998

[20] Salem AA, Shakel EA, Sadakha AA, Kassem EM, El-Segai AA. Evaluation of Zygomatic implant retained obturator in rehabilitation of partial palato-maxillectomy patients. Tanta Dental Journal. 2015;**12**(1):35-40. DOI: 10.1016/j.tdj.2014.10.003

[21] Rosenstein J, Dym H. Zygomatic implants: A solution for the atrophic maxilla. Dental Clinics of North America. 2020;**64**(2):401-409. DOI: 10.1016/j.cden.2019.12.005

[22] King E, Abbott C, Dovgalski L, Owens J. Orofacial rehabilitation with zygomatic implants: CAD-CAM bar and magnets for patients with nasal cancer after rhinectomy and partial maxillectomy. Journal of Prosthetic Dentistry. 2017;**117**(6):806-810. DOI: 10.1016/j.prosdent.2016.09.029

[23] Aparicio C, Ouazzani W, Hatano N. The use of zygomatic implants for prosthetic rehabilitation of the severely resorbed maxilla. Periodontology 2000. 2000;**47**(1):162-171

[24] Tulasne JF. Implant treatment of missing posterior dentition. In: Albrektson T, Zarb G, editors. The Branemark Osseointegrated Implant. Chicago: Quintessence; 1989. p. 103-115

[25] Bidra AS, Huynh-Ba G. Implants in the pterygoid region: A systematic review of the literature. International Journal of Oral and Maxillofacial Surgery. 2011;**40**(8):773-781. DOI: 10.1016/j.ijom.2011.04.007

[26] Araujo RZ, Santiago Júnior JF, Cardoso CL, Benites Condezo AF, Moreira Júnior R, Curi MM. Clinical outcomes of pterygoid implants: Systematic review and meta-analysis. Journal of Cranio-Maxillofacial Surgery. 2019;**47**(4):651-660. DOI: 10.1016/j.jcms.2019.01.030

[27] Schepers RH, Slagter AP, Kaanders JHAM, van den Hoogen FJA, Merkx MAW. Effect of postoperative radiotherapy on the functional result of implants placed during ablative surgery for oral cancer. International Journal of Oral and Maxillofacial Surgery. 2006;**35**(9):803-808

[28] Okay DJ, Genden E, Buchbinder D, Urken M. Prosthodontic guidelines for surgical reconstruction of the maxilla. The Journal of Prosthetic Dentistry. 2001;**86**(4):352-363

[29] Surovas A. A digital workflow for modeling of custom dental implants. 3D

Printing in Medicine. 2019;**5**(9):01-11. DOI: 10.1186/s41205-019-0046-y

[30] Wentaschek S, Lehmann K, Scheller H, Weibrich G, Behneke N. Polygonal area of prosthesis support with straight and tilted dental implants in edentulous maxillae. The International Journal of Prosthodontics. 2016;**29**(3):245-252

[31] Raman R, Bashir R. Stereolithographic 3D bioprinting for biomedical applications. In: Essentials of 3D Biofabrication and Translation. Elsevier Inc.; 2015. pp. 89-121. DOI: 10.1016/B978-0-12-800972-7/00006-2

[32] Martelli N, Serrano C, Van Den Brink H, Pineau J, Prognon P, Borget I, et al. Advantages and disadvantages of 3-dimensional printing in surgery: A systematic review. Surgery. 2016;**159**(6):1485-1500

[33] Garritano FG, Fedok F. Facial reconstruction after resection for cutaneous malignancies. Operative Techniques in Otolaryngology. 2013;**24**(1):36-44. DOI: 10.1016/j.otot.2013.03.002

[34] Unkovskiy A, Spintzyk S, Brom J, Huettig F, Keutel C. Direct 3D printing of silicone facial prostheses: A preliminary experience in digital workflow. Journal of Prosthetic Dentistry. 2018;**120**(2):303-308. DOI: 10.1016/j.prosdent.2017.11.007

[35] McHutchion L, Aalto D. Simulation of tissue-prosthesis margin interface by using surface scanning and digital design for auricular prostheses. Journal of Prosthetic Dentistry. 2020:1-12. DOI: 10.1016/j.prosdent.2020.01.045

[36] Ellis MA, Graboyes EM, Wahlquist AE, Neskey DM, Kaczmar JM, Schopper HK, et al. Primary surgery vs. radiotherapy for early stage oral cavity cancer. Otolaryngology–Head and Neck Surgery. 2018;**158**(4):649-659

[37] Brennan PA, Bradley KL, Brands M. Intensity-modulated radiotherapy in head and neck cancer — An update for oral and maxillofacial surgeons. British Journal of Oral and Maxillofacial Surgery. 2017;**55**(8):770-774. DOI: 10.1016/j.bjoms.2017.07.019

[38] Schiegnitz E, Al-Nawas B, Kämmerer PW, Grötz KA. Oral rehabilitation with dental implants in irradiated patients: A meta-analysis on implant survival. Clinical Oral Investigations. 2014;**18**(3):687-698

[39] Zen Filho EV, Tolentino EDS, Santos PSS. Viability of dental implants in head and neck irradiated patients: A systematic review. Head & Neck. 2016;**38**:E2229–E2240

[40] Granados M, Arrieta O, Cantú de León D. Oncología y cirugía. In: Bases y principios. 1a ed. México: Manual Moderno; 2013. p. 768. Available from: https://books.google.com/books?id=xWTLCQAAQBAJ&pgis=1

[41] Al-Jandan B, Marei HF, Abuohashish H, Zakaria O, Al-Mahalawy H. Effects of sunitinib targeted chemotherapy on the osseointegration of titanium implants. Biomedicine & Pharmacotherapy. 2018;**100**(January):433-440

[42] Al-Jandan B, Marei HF, Abuohashish H, Zakaria O, Al-Mahalawy H. Effects of cisplatin chemotherapy on the osseointegration of titanium implants. Biomedicine & Pharmacotherapy. 2018;**100**:433-440

[43] Al-Jandan B. Effect of antiangiogenic targeted chemotherapy on the osseointegration of titanium implants in rabbits. The British Journal of Oral & Maxillofacial Surgery. 2019;**57**(2):157-163

[44] Javed F, Al-Hezaimi K, Al-Rasheed A, Almas K, Romanos GE. Implant survival rate after oral cancer therapy: A review. Oral Oncology.

2010;**46**(12):854-859. DOI: 10.1016/j.oraloncology.2010.10.004

[45] Kovács AF. Influence of chemotherapy on endosteal implant survival and success in oral cancer patients. International Journal of Oral and Maxillofacial Surgery. 2001;**30**(2):144-147

[46] Kovács AF. The fate of osseointegrated implants in patients following oral cancer surgery and mandibular reconstruction. Head & Neck. 2000;**22**(2):111-119